P9-CEC-527

PRAISE FOR

Naturally Sweet and Gluten-Free

"*Naturally Sweet* is not only a visual delight, its recipes are amazing, too! I've come to rely on the fluffy pancakes and the oat muffins as staples, and plan to work my way through every healthy indulgence one goodie at a time."   —Alisa Marie Fleming, author of *Go Dairy Free*

"In this gorgeous book, Ricki Heller shows people with dietary concerns how they, too, can enjoy decadent desserts. It is solid proof that a seemingly restrictive style of eating can, in fact, be an absolute joy!"
—Allyson Kramer, author of *Sweet Eats for All* and
Great Gluten-Free Vegan Eats

"Talk about tempting! Chocolate Pecan Pie and Butterscotch–Chocolate Chip Cookies? Yes please! . . . This book needs to be on your shelf!"   —Kathy Patalsky, author of *365 Vegan Smoothies*

"Once in a while a cookbook comes along that is a game-changer. Opening its pages may introduce a new dietary approach or cuisine that forever shifts our food choices. Or, perhaps opening that book enables us to reintroduce foods we used to love, but we thought we could never delight in again because of dietary needs. Ricki Heller's newly released *Naturally Sweet & Gluten-Free* is exactly this kind of game-changing book. If you love to make sweets but want to bake cleaner, with whole-grains, no sugar, and also avoiding allergens like gluten and corn, this book will open a whole new world of baking for you. If you are already eating a plant-based/vegan/gluten-free/low-glycemic diet, you will think you are dreaming when you open this book! Ricki is making your dessert dreams come true! Go ahead and do your happy dance because you can have your gluten-free, vegan, and sugar-free cake . . . and eat it, too!"

—Dreena Burton, author of *Let Them Eat Vegan!*

Living Candida-Free

ALSO BY RICKI HELLER

Naturally Sweet & Gluten-Free:
Allergy-Friendly Vegan Desserts: 100 Recipes Without
Gluten, Dairy, Eggs, or Refined Sugar

Sweet Freedom: Desserts You'll Love Without
Wheat, Eggs, Dairy, or Refined Sugar

LIVING CANDIDA-FREE

*100 Recipes and a
3-Stage Program
to Restore Your
Health and Vitality*

RICKI HELLER, PhD, RHN

with Andrea Nakayama, CNC, CNE, CHHC

Da Capo
LIFE
LONG

A Member of the Perseus Books Group

Copyright © 2015 by Ricki Heller
Photos by Nicole Axworthy

Note that the following recipe was cocreated by Andrea Nakayama and chef Andrea Livingston for their TrulyFood Cleanse series. Used by permission.
Almost Instant Grain-Free Breakfast Porridge (page 127)

All rights reserved. No part of this publication may be reproduced, stored in a retrieval system, or transmitted, in any form or by any means, electronic, mechanical, photocopying, recording, or otherwise, without the prior written permission of the publisher. Printed in the United States of America. For information, address Da Capo Press, 44 Farnsworth Street, 3rd Floor, Boston, MA 02210

Designed by Timm Bryson
Set in 11 point Warnock Pro by the Perseus Books Group

Library of Congress Cataloging-in-Publication Data

Heller, Ricki.
  Living candida-free: 100 recipes and a 3-phase program to restore your health and vitality / Ricki Heller, PHD, RHN ; with Andrea Nakayama, CNC, CNE, CHHC.
     pages cm
  Includes bibliographical references and index.
  ISBN 978-0-7382-1775-8 (paperback) — ISBN 978-0-7382-1776-5 (e-book) 1. Candidiasis—Diet therapy—Recipes. 2. Yeast-free diet—Recipes. I. Nakayama, Andrea. II. Title.

  RC123.C3H47 2015
  641.5'63—dc23
                    2014036261

First Da Capo Press edition 2015

Published by Da Capo Press
A Member of the Perseus Books Group
www.dacapopress.com

Note: The information in this book is true and complete to the best of our knowledge. This book is intended only as an informative guide for those wishing to know more about health issues. In no way is this book intended to replace, countermand, or conflict with the advice given to you by your own physician. The ultimate decision concerning care should be made between you and your doctor. We strongly recommend you follow his or her advice. Information in this book is general and is offered with no guarantees on the part of the authors or Da Capo Press. The authors and publisher disclaim all liability in connection with the use of this book.

Da Capo Press books are available at special discounts for bulk purchases in the U.S. by corporations, institutions, and other organizations. For more information, please contact the Special Markets Department at the Perseus Books Group, 2300 Chestnut Street, Suite 200, Philadelphia, PA, 19103, or call (800) 810-4145, ext. 5000, or e-mail special.markets@perseusbooks.com.

10 9 8 7 6 5 4 3 2 1

This book is dedicated to my mom,
who would have benefited immensely from it.

CONTENTS

CHAPTER 11: Salads, Dressings, and Sauces 163

CHAPTER 12: Mains 183

INTRODUCTION

Once you choose hope, anything's possible.
—CHRISTOPHER REEVE

Do you sometimes feel as if there's a war going on inside your body, and—even though you never enlisted—you're the one losing the battle? Your body is fighting a stealthy adversary that seems to be everywhere at once: you may be suffering from IBS (irritable bowel syndrome), get recurrent sinus infections, have chronic yeast infections or rashes, or experience general malaise. These are only some of the symptoms of candida. Or perhaps you've noticed what are the most common symptoms of candida: overwhelming cravings for sugars or carbs and a feeling of spaciness or "fuzzy thinking," so that getting your mind to focus on a single thing can seem impossible.

No wonder so many people with candida-related complex (CRC, or, simply, "candida") feel discouraged and may even begin to despair, when doctors can't seem to pinpoint what's wrong and nothing seems to make it better.

Well, I'm here to tell you: there is hope, and you *can* heal. Yes, candida is a formidable opponent, but, with diligence and the right approach, it's possible to get it under control and restore your health. In my case, I had an exceptionally severe and stubborn case of candida-related complex, and I was able to heal and get better. In fact, my health improved beyond what it was *before* the candida.

In this book, I'm going to tell you how I did it—and what you can do, too.

My Story

I found myself at the dermatologist's office again, the fifth time in three months. The raw, raging rash on my torso wasn't getting any smaller; if anything, it was growing. I'd been following a strict no-sugar, no-yeast diet for eight weeks, and I'd tried every prescription cream the doctor could think of. I'd just completed a two-week course of Diflucan, a powerful antifungal pill, which was the only thing that seemed to make any dent at all, helping reduce the unbearable itch that plagued me every waking moment. Now, the doctor was telling me she wouldn't prescribe a second course of the pills.

"It can't be candida," she said, the way you'd speak to a tourist asking for directions. "It would be gone after two weeks with those pills if it were candida. Try alternating the Canesten cream with some zinc oxide ointment. . . . "

I began to sob inconsolably. "Please, you have to help me. It's spreading," I insisted.

"Diflucan is the only thing that had any effect at all. *Just look at it.*" I pointed to the angry crimson splotch the size of a Stop sign. Blistering, crusty edges surrounded an amorphous red patch dotted with areas of tender pink flesh. "The itching finally stopped when I took the Diflucan. All I'm asking is two more weeks. One of the books that I've been reading says—"

"I will not give you more Diflucan," she barked, cutting me off. "If the Diflucan didn't clear it up yet, it's never going to clear it up. Okay, now. Just keep using the cream and the zinc oxide. . . . " She turned toward the door. "Come back in a few weeks and we'll take another look."

"In a few weeks, it will have covered my entire body if you don't do something," I said, as the door shut behind her.

Sadly, my experience with that dermatologist—the fourth doctor I'd seen in search of some answers about my candida-related complex—is not atypical. And let me be clear: this woman was a conscientious physician who truly wanted to help her patients; she just had no context for treating me.

I knew beyond a doubt that my problems were somehow related to candida, and I knew from its effect that the prescription antifungal was essential to mitigate its growth. But back then, in 2009—and to a great extent, still today—conventional medicine didn't accept "candida" as a real medical condition.

How did I get to that point? How could I, someone trained as a holistic nutritionist and armed with all the necessary knowledge about the perils of sugar—someone who'd actually studied nutrition as a direct result of symptoms related to candida ten years earlier—how did I end up with one of the most resistant cases of candida-related complex my naturopath had ever seen?

A Sugar Addict from Day One

Anyone who feels powerless in the face of a chocolate brownie likely already knows this, but only recently has science concurred with the notion that sugar is addictive. Such best-selling books as Mark Hyman's *The Blood Sugar Solution*[1] or David Kessler's *The End of Overeating*[2] discuss at length the special addictive properties of the white stuff. For me, sugar was always the drug of choice.

Almost as soon as I could walk, I could bake. At age six I began to help my mother in the kitchen, spending entire afternoons studying her culinary prowess as she stirred up huge bowls of cookie dough, blended cottage cheese with eggs and lemon for my dad's favorite cheesecake, or whipped egg whites until triple in volume for her famous chiffon cake. At each step along the way, I might help by contributing a cup of flour or a sprinkling of chocolate chips, but, for me, by far the best part was after the batter was in the oven and I could lick the spoon or beaters, or scrape the bowl clean. My sisters and I would regularly bicker over who got which utensil.

In retrospect, it's clear that I began to manifest symptoms of candida even back then. Shortly after our first dog, a sweet boxer named Princess, began to share my bed, I was diagnosed with ringworm, an itchy scarlet rash across the hairline at the back of my neck. It was attributed to the dog, of course, and, with a bit of ointment, it disappeared—or so I assumed. It wasn't until years later that I learned ringworm is actually a form of fungus and was most likely an augury of the more intense candida-related rash to come down the road.

The love affair with sweets continued through my teens and twenties. As the "responsible daughter," I was always left in charge of my younger sister when my parents went on vacation. As soon as their taxi drove out of sight, my sister and I threw on our jackets and headed to the supermarket. There, I'd spend the entire week's grocery money stocking up for our weekend "party": we filled the cart with every kind of junk food imaginable, from tubs of Heavenly Hash ice cream to family-size milk chocolate bars and boxes of fudge-filled sandwich cookies . . . in other words, whatever was normally forbidden in our "homemade only" household. As soon as the bags were loaded and the groceries paid for, we'd head home, settle down on my parents' bed in front of the TV, and proceed to devour the entire haul.

Candida, Take One

By the time I reached my thirties and got married, I was beset with recurrent yeast infections that no one could explain—or cure. I wasn't officially diagnosed with candida, however, until later in that decade, when I'd suffered a series of recurring sinus infections that finally became so severe that, after six courses of antibiotics, I spiked a 104°F (40°C) fever. That day, I'd been to yet another physician who could do nothing but prescribe more drugs. My husband had taken off work because I was too sick to drive to the doctor's office on my own. When we arrived home, I was depressed, despondent, and so weak that I literally was unable to walk up the stairs to our bedroom and had to crawl up step-by-step on my hands and knees. At that point, it finally hit me: something major had to change (yes, I'm a little thick-headed that way).

Luckily, I stumbled upon a holistically minded doctor who recognized my condition and started me on a course of nystatin (an antifungal drug) along with a strict anticandida diet (ACD). I followed her regimen to the letter for two years and ultimately considered myself entirely "cured" of my condition. The ACD I followed back then included mostly vegetables, fish, and eggs, with no sugars, fruit, fungi, alcohol, or fermented foods. During that time, I attended the Canadian School of Natural Nutrition as well, where I learned about the *whys* of candida in addition to more about the diet. Now that I was surrounded by like-minded individuals and holistic health professionals, that year marked a high point in my health: the sinus infections disappeared, I felt great, and I turned to a healthy, vegan, whole foods diet. I continued to consume only whole foods ingredients, with no refined sugars or flours; my sweeteners of choice were natural alternatives, such as maple syrup, dates, or Sucanat (unrefined cane sugar).

During that interval, in fact, my health issues all but vanished. I not only stopped taking medication I'd been on for hypothyroidism, but I was also able to wean off medication I'd been taking for sixteen years for my irritable bowel syndrome (IBS). As long as I ate real, whole foods and used natural sweeteners, I seemed to be fine. Life was never better.

As my body continued to thrive for the next decade, inevitably, I became a little too cocky about my health and began to resume some of my previous eating habits. In no time, I was once again consuming the selfsame offending foods that had got me in trouble in the first place, from sugar- and refined flour–laden baked goods to glasses of wine with dinner to favorite junk foods.

Within a matter of months, I noticed a dime-size rash on my chest. Unwilling to accept that it could be candida returning, I ignored it until it grew to the size of a quarter. But when it started to spread beyond the boundaries of my bra, I couldn't overlook it any longer; within a month or so, I was in a dermatologist's office, where she prescribed Canesten cream, confirming that it was, indeed, a fungal rash.

Only this time, the simple treatment didn't work. I knew that I should return to the diet that had been so instrumental in conquering candida the first time but was loathe to give up all the food indulgences I'd so recently brought back into my life. Before too long, the rash had spread down my torso. I wandered from one dermatologist to the next, each one prescribing a different cream, but none could eradicate the rash.

By the time I was bawling in that last dermatologist's office, I could almost see the rash growing in real time, like an ink stain spreading out on a favorite sweater.

Candida, Take Two

My second experience with candida was so much worse than the first that it truly changed my life. I'm no longer certain that any change is "forever," but I do believe that the diet and lifestyle I now follow are so fully entrenched as habits that there is little chance of a recurrence. At this point, I've both experienced and studied the condition enough that I've amassed a great deal of knowledge, both firsthand through academic study as well as through the hundreds of comments and e-mails I receive daily from readers of my blog and books. I could never have imagined when I began my blog back in 2009 that it would become the source of information, guidance, and comfort to hundreds of thousands of visitors that it is today. To paraphrase Shakespeare, having had this form of expertise "thrust upon" me, I now willingly embrace it.

These days, I live my life fully but never forget my experience with candida. I hold a new respect for the power of fungus and mold in our lives and know that the balance between "well" and "ill" can be precarious. I still enjoy desserts, chocolate, baked goods, bread, pasta, and many other foods that I thought I'd have to give up forever. But the difference is that nowadays, my definition of *binge* is eating perhaps four homemade raw cookie dough truffles (recipe on page 209) instead of an entire batch in one sitting. It doesn't mean that I don't still desire the whole batch (sometimes I do), but I know that kind of overindulgence could very well lead to a situation in which my candida might once more overtake my health, so I stop before that can happen.

I continue to learn how to listen to my body and honor what it needs. And I know, as long as I travel down this path, while still enjoying a plethora of delicious food, my body will repay me with a vibrant health, wellness, and a strong immune system. I wish the same for you, too.

What's in It for You/How to Use This Book

If you're reading this book, you're likely feeling a certain degree of urgency in your own search for answers. You may feel sick, weak, and desperate for someone to tell you what to do to feel better *right now*. At that moment in the dermatologist's office, had someone promised me, "Leave your husband forever and I'll get rid of it for you," well, I would have had to really think about it. (Don't worry; the dogs were still safe.)

This book is designed to share with you the steps I took to gain control of my own severe case of CRC and to learn to live my life with a renewed sense of freedom and wellness. After following an anticandida lifestyle for more than fifteen years, these days, I'm delighted to be able to help others who may be going through similar situations.

As a registered holistic nutritionist and educator, I speak at conferences, work with companies, and teach courses on balancing blood sugar and successfully navigating the anticandida diet. As a blogger at rickiheller.com, I offer readers information, online programs, and support; as a freelance writer and magazine editor, I create recipes, conduct research, and write articles about healthy, vegan, gluten-free, and lower-glycemic foods.

But perhaps more important, I now have all the energy I need for those sixteen-hour workdays, I exercise regularly, I spend time with my husband and beloved dogs—in other words, I live a pretty normal, productive life—and 99 percent of the time, I forget that I ever had candida. Even when I followed the early, stricter form of the diet for several years, I didn't let that stop me from socializing with friends and family, or traveling, or taking vacations. Yes, it can be done!

Still, just like recovered alcoholics who continue to label themselves as such, I will always have candida, and, if I'm not careful, I know it may resurface at any time.

Depending on the severity of the condition, that will certainly not be the case for everyone; many people with less severe levels of candida infestation recover fully and never have to worry about eating sugar, drinking alcohol, or consuming moldy foods (e.g., peanuts) or edible fungi (e.g., mushrooms) again. I just know that's not me.

Because I am neither a doctor nor a scientist, this book is not designed to provide you with a definitive diagnosis or minute details about the biochemistry of *Candida albicans* (although functional nutritionist Andrea Nakayama does a splendid job with that topic in Chapter 1). I won't share reams of scientific studies that prove or disprove the existence of candida-related complex or require a medical degree to understand.

What you'll find here instead is a *practical approach* that helps you understand the origin and progression of candida in the body; a comprehensive means to assess for yourself whether you suffer from the condition (plus other tests your health-care practitioner can order); and realistic, achievable steps you can take to get the candida under control in a way that won't prevent you from living your "real" life.

Healing will take a different route for each one of us, depending on the severity and causes of our condition, so this is not a hard-and-fast prescription for how to cure candida-related complex.

In this book, my aim is to provide you with feasible, easily implemented strategies and techniques so you'll not only adhere successfully to your anticandida diet but will also thrive and even enjoy yourself as you do so.

This is a pragmatic guidebook for anyone just diagnosed with CRC or about to start an anticandida diet. If you've been battling the beast that is yeast for some time and are looking for a new approach that will actually work, this book is for you, too. It's for you, as well, if you feel that sugar plays too powerful a role in your life and you'd like to remove it entirely, or lower the overall glycemic load of foods you eat. I encourage you to work with your health-care practitioner and use your own body's reactions and responses to help you design the perfect anticandida diet *for you*, working within the general guidelines of this book.

The techniques in this book don't require that you eat the exact diet I followed. Although my recipes are vegan, the guidelines here allow anyone, vegan or omnivore, to succeed at beating candida. I'll show you how to cook food that tastes delicious and that you'll be happy to serve to family and friends (so you don't have to cook two dinners every night). I've served Eggplant "Parmesan" (page 192) and Sunday Night Roast with Perfect Golden Gravy (page 196 and 177) to family and friends alike, and everyone has loved them. Chocolate-Covered Chocolate Chip Cookie Dough Truffles (page 209–210) or Grain-Free Apple Berry Crumble (page 212) with Vanilla Ice Cream (page 220) make a great finish to any meal, anticandida diet–friendly or not. I'll also help you revamp some of your old recipes to render them ACD-compliant, and how to clean up and monitor your home so you don't encourage yeast to grow in your personal environment. And most important, I'll show you that it's entirely possible to do more than merely survive while following an anticandida diet.

Yes, your journey will be challenging at times and it may require more planning around food than you're used to. But it's entirely achievable, and, in very little time, living a life without sugar or yeast that is happy, fulfilling, and healthy will begin to feel like second nature.

Before we get into the actual diet protocol, you'll hear from Andrea Nakayama. Andrea is a functional nutritionist who specializes in awakening personal transformation through educating both clients and practitioners in the science and physiology of nutrition. In Chapter 1, she provides a science-based overview of what the heck candida is, how it grows, and why it wreaks such havoc on the body. We've also included a Yeast Assessment form (see page 236) to help you determine your own best course of action.

After you've got a sound basis for CRC, we'll jump into the overview of the ACD, followed by detailed information on the different stages of the diet. You'll learn which foods should go on your grocery list and which you should toss in the trash, plus some simple tricks for converting your favorite foods to ACD-friendly fare. And, of course, there are the recipes: one hundred easy, flavorful dishes. You'll find basics, such as nut milks and nut butters; simple sauces and condiments; hearty breakfasts; sides and snacks; quick and easy lunches and soups; salads and dressings; and satisfying mains. And while you might be dreading a sugar-free life, you can indulge, too, with some of my amazing sweet treats. If you're keen to examine the diet plan, go ahead to Chapter 2; if you'd rather just start by sampling some of the book's recipes, those begin in Chapter 6.

Part I

What Is Candida— and What Can I Do About It?

CHAPTER 1

Candida-Related Complex: What It Is, How It Develops, and How to Get a Proper Diagnosis

by Andrea Nakayama, CNC, CHE, CHHC

You've likely picked up this book because your body demands to know what's going on and how it can get better. Congratulations for taking the proactive step to manage your health yourself. Diet and lifestyle are key ways in which we step back into the driver's seat and take ownership of our well-being. It's not always easy and you may be fed up by now, having tried various tactics to feel better, yet I know you'll soon relish the empowering feelings of knowing *how to deal* and *how to heal*.

Your symptoms might be fleeting and intangible, such as fatigue, memory loss, brain fog, or depression. Conversely, you might have physical proof of imbalance with diarrhea, constipation, headache, rashes, hives, or eczema.

You might be sensitive to foods you love to eat, but you don't want to stop eating them. Or you may have lost interest in eating altogether because, let's face it, nothing seems to feel good or rest well in your belly. These cries for help are specific signals from various organs and internal systems demanding attention and alternative action.

3

When you learn the language of those cries for help, harmony and connection can and will occur. As with any relationship, the one you're about to develop with your own self may come with challenges. This crucial step you're taking in educating yourself about your health and deepening your awareness of your signs and symptoms will help put you on the path to recovery. When you've finished reading this chapter, you'll know far more about the body than your average human. You'll also have the opportunity to *feel better* than the average adult, a state of being that has seemed to evade you for far too long. Take a deep breath; liberation is within reach.

My Journey to Health

As a functional nutritionist, I've helped hundreds of individual clients and thousands of online (cleanse and detox) participants regain their health through education and knowledge. Understanding imbalance puts everything into context.

My own road to nutrition grew out of a curiosity that was honed in the face of a family health crisis. In April 2000 my husband was diagnosed with a fatal brain tumor and given six months to live. I was seven weeks pregnant with our first and only child at the time. My husband died when our son, Gilbert, was nineteen months old, over two years after his diagnosis.

It was during that period that I discovered food was not only something that I loved to explore at the farmers' market, prepare in my kitchen, and savor on my plate but also a substance that could have powerful healing benefits. Food and diet empowered me to make a difference—in my husband's life (extending it well beyond the prognosis), in my son's life, in the communities I serve online, and now in yours. Initially this focus on diet and nutrition gave me something I could do every day, several times a day, to nurture my growing family. Now, with the extensive training I've gone through since that time, I'm able to help propose the root cause of illnesses and address the appropriate diet to suit the needs of the underlying condition. The key is the diet, but the lock is your unique physiology—at the level of your genes, your cells, and your organ function, particularly your gut, as we're going to explore.

The gut and digestive system are at the core of almost every health challenge. For myself, the constitution of my gastrointestinal (GI) tract is a prime focus in the management of my autoimmune thyroid condition (called Hashimoto's thyroiditis). For you, in handling candida and the many signs, symptoms, and even diagnosis that can be triggered by this condition, it really does come back to the seat of digestion.

You Are What You Eat . . . or Are You?

To begin, let's reframe an important belief: You are not what you eat; rather, you are what your body can *do* with what you eat. In other words, you are what your body can break down and absorb, what you do and do not eliminate. In many ways you are also the sum of your parts. You are likely aware of the usual digestive parts—your mouth and esophagus, your stomach and intestines—but your digestive system is also host to a vast number of bacteria, protozoa, and fungi. Candida is one of those fungi.

The human body is made up of about 10 trillion cells. Yet there are approximately ten times as many microorganisms living right within your intestines. In fact, it's your gut and other mucous membranes, such as your respiratory or urogenital tract, that create a home for those bacteria, protozoa, and fungi.

This part of your body, called your microbiome, consists of trillions of tiny microbes often referred to as microflora—single-celled organisms that are so minuscule that millions can fit in the eye of a needle. These different kinds of microorganisms are all designed to live in a symbiotic and nonharmful relationship with *you*. (Note that the words *microbiome*, *microflora*, and *microbiota* are often used interchangeably.)

There's really nothing to be grossed out about when thinking of sharing your body with these tiny organisms. It's natural, normal. In fact, these little organisms do quite a lot to keep you alive and enable you to thrive. They help you train your immune system, prevent the growth of harmful bacteria that can make you sick, create a barrier from exposure to all sorts of agents that you come into contact with every day, produce antibiotic-like substances that are antifungal and antiviral, regulate the growth and development of the gastrointestinal tract, produce vitamins for you, and even manufacture certain hormones. (Instead of being grossed out, we should thank these little critters!)

There has been an increasing amount of research, clinical studies, and investigation into the role of the microbiome on our health. Some of this inquiry has focused on our immune system and how our bodies protect us from foreigners at the microscopic level. Other analysis has been in relation to the connection between the gut and the brain, whether that be its maturation, mood, or motivation. Bacterial analysis has looked at the composition of microflora in connection to heart health, weight management, and complexion. Perhaps most curiously, newer research shows that what you eat interacts, not only with *you*, but also with your flora. The food we eat can change the makeup and function of our gut microbiome for the good or for the bad.

You are not just what you eat, but what your body and your biome can do with what you eat!

Mapping Your Microbiome

Most of the flora and their concomitant organisms take residence in your colon. The largest populations of organisms that dwell there tend to be bacterial, as opposed to the protozoa or fungi that may also inhabit the terrain. Yet this is where we all differ. Although you and I both have a colon (unless, of course, it's been surgically removed), the culture and populace of your flora is likely very different than mine. For instance, an overburdened bacterial population in your microbiome may have allowed for a yeast overgrowth, whereas I may have a proliferation of a certain type of bacterium, throwing my flora out of balance (and setting the stage for my autoimmune imbalance). There will also be a variance between the bacterial composition in each and every one of us at the most basic level, between the good and the bad—the commensal and the opportunistic.

A significant number of factors throughout your life will affect the composition of your flora, starting before birth. That's just the beginning. Your microflora grows and morphs from there, throughout your life. Other factors that will influence your microflora population include:

- type of delivery
- immunizations
- breast or bottle feeding
- use of antibiotics or other pharmaceuticals, such as birth control pills, steroids, or hormone replacement therapy
- chemotherapy or radiation
- diet
- drug or alcohol use
- stress

- location within the body (e.g., vaginal bacteria is different than the bacteria in the mouth)
- geographical environment
- age
- overall health and immune status

It's even been shown that, within the same individual factors such as hormonal fluctuations, dietary changes, abrupt shifts in stress levels, and sexual activity can cause alterations in the population of the microflora.

I draw this all out to provide you with some context. It's sometimes hard to understand why your roommate or spouse or best friend can eat a hot fudge sundae without experiencing immediate fatigue, brain fog, and bloating. Or why it is that your sister doesn't suffer chronic health challenges, such as persistent skin irritations and anal itching, sustained upper respiratory infections, anxiety, and fibroids, even though she stops for a jumbo chocolate chip cookie on the way back to the office from lunch *every* single day. When it comes to candida, context is everything—the context in which the yeast within you has to grow.

In many ways, our health boils down to that microscopic internal environment and the ways in which yours is unique to you in this very moment. Your flora is like the sum of your experiences. You've collected a little of this, a lot of that; you've distributed some of your organisms and unknowingly exterminated others. What you carry inside your gut is a recipe that you and only you could have created. But you certainly aren't the only one who has established an environment that's ripe for the growth of candida.

Candida Doesn't Discriminate

Candida has gotten a lot more attention in the last decade or so, and with good reason. As noted earlier, candida—specifically, *Candida albicans*—is a yeast, a kind of fungus. We've always had some of the yeast present in our bodies at any one time, and everybody has some—regardless of age or gender. Candida doesn't discriminate. And candida isn't the problem; the environment is.

In a healthy person, candida is a harmless agent. Yet fluctuations in the internal bacterial environment that influence immune health enable the yeast to grow past its tipping point, past the point where its actions are kept in check by the host climate. In these circumstances, the same harmless strains of candida can become pathogenic, invading the mucosa and causing significant damage.

Candida is an intelligent and networked organism. It's considered a dimorphic fungus—meaning it can change shapes, oscillating between a bud and hyphae (the latter looking more like a little sperm), depending on its surrounding habitat. *Dimorphic* literally means "with two shapes." It's the longer filaments, the hyphae, that can burrow their roots through the mucosal barriers and into your tissues to initiate so-called leaky gut—a situation where one of the body's most important boundaries and barricades between the inside and outside world has been breached. Without suitable restraint, any number of elements, including improperly broken-down constituents from the food you've eaten, can make their way into your bloodstream and wreak further havoc on your health. This may appear as inflammation, allergies, asthma, eczema, food intolerances, headaches, joint pain, and mind challenges, such as depression, anxiety, mood swings, and problems with memory or focus.

Within a suitably compromised mucosal atmosphere, candida is tailored to gain power and proliferate. The environment that will support its growth is one where there's a lot of undigested sugar and starch for it to feed on as well as a climate that has a lower pH, meaning that it is more acidic. Sugar, starches, and simple carbohydrates in the diet contribute to both of these generative factors, which is why diet is such an important part of an anticandida protocol—and why we've put together this food-based plan for you.

Because the yeast is a part of the microflora lodged in the mucosa, and much of this mucosa is situated in the gut, we're brought right back to my very first belief: you are not what you eat, but what your body can *do* with what you eat. When a favorable environment for yeast overgrowth exists in the microflora, then what you do with that pie à la mode is make more yeast. And as you make more yeast, you put more strain on your immune system to try to gain back some balance. This leaves you tired and inflamed and can cause confusion among your immune cells as they try to discern "self" from "other."

As the yeast "feeds" on the sugars in its environment, it begs for more. It's like a growing child. *Its* need for more sugars manifests as *your* sweet tooth. I like to remind my clients that what feels like a lack of willpower when trying to avoid sweets or carbohydrates may be something much more sovereign to contend with—a growing and hungry pathogen.

As the yeast feeds it also metabolizes. The by-products left behind from the yeasts' feast are perhaps more dangerous to your health than the yeast itself. These are toxic chemicals and dead yeast cells classified as mycotoxins (little fungal poisons) that can be released into your bloodstream. Some of these will undoubtedly leave you feeling fuzzy and hungover; others can interfere with your body's abilities to produce key antioxidants and suppress the function of your immune system by thwarting the production of white blood cells.

The Key to CRC: Become an Environmentalist

Thinking about candida through the lens of its offenses can be overwhelming. And yet it doesn't have to be. This is where you get to become an environmentalist so you can learn to alter the habitat within you and make it one that is less hospitable to candida overgrowth and more conducive to balance.

Let's look at the environment of your digestive system, top to bottom, and uncover exactly what its two major functions—*digest* and *absorb*—actually mean, so that we can look at how a yeast overgrowth affects its performance and how that, in turn, affects *you*.

Your Digestive Superhighway

Food is the carrier for microscopic nutrition. Microscopic nutrition is essentially the minute chemical components of your food. The digestive system is the highway along which that microscopic nutrition travels, and your cells are the final destination. What this means is that not only is your diet fundamental, so is the health of your digestive superhighway. The relationship between how and what you eat, how you can process what you eat, and ultimately how you feel is undeniable—especially in relation to CRC.

There are several ways in which the inside of your body interacts with the outside world. Between the two (inside and outside), you have what are called barrier systems. They're designed to protect you. Your barrier systems include your skin and those mucous membranes that house the microflora, and that are found in the obvious areas, such as your nose and mouth, as well as throughout your digestive, respiratory, and genitourinary tracts. The constituents that interact with and bypass these protective barriers make their way into your bloodstream to interact with every cell in your body.

These constituents consist of those minute chemical components from the food you eat as well as those myriad microbes, yeasts, and pathogens. (Oh my!)

I've seen the digestive system likened to a donut. If you visualize this, you can appreciate that the hole of the donut is separate from the donut itself, right? The two are separate from each other. Yet, while the digestive system is essentially separate from the rest of the body, everything that travels through that digestive tract—spanning from your mouth to your anus—interacts with your inside world as well. Various mechanisms allow for this interaction, some in support of your best health and others that become factors in your ill health. Taking a journey through the digestive superhighway—the pathway for the food to transform into the micronutrients that we need at a cellular level—will help refine our understanding of why, what, and where things might go off path, especially as relates to candida overgrowth and how this might be affecting your health.

The word *nutrient* means a nutritive substance, something that is there to nourish, support growth, maintain the body, and to repair what might need fixing. Proteins, as we'll see through our travels, are broken down into peptides, which are digested (broken down) into amino acids, which are absorbed at the level of the small intestine to get into the bloodstream and feed your cells. Carbohydrates are digested into monosaccharides, such as glucose, fructose, and galactose, which are also absorbed at the level of the small intestine so they can go into the bloodstream and also be fed to your cells. Fats are digested into fatty acids and absorbed in the small intestine, again, to feed your hungry cells. These three nutrients—proteins, carbohydrates, and fats—make up our macronutrients, the things we need to consume to survive. Your cells need food, too. Their food just comes in a different package. Digestion is the technique that transforms your food to your cell's fuel.

Digestion is one of the essential jobs of the human body. It's a cascade of actions whereby the success of each event is considerably dependent on the completion of the prior action. Throughout the digestive system are two means by which the food on your plate is converted into the microscopic nutrient that feeds your cells. Those two means consist of a mechanical and a chemical breakdown. It's by both of these methods that we create those amino acids, simple sugars, and fatty acids out of a turkey or tempeh sandwich (and out of their proteins, fats, and carbohydrates). When it comes to food, you can think of yourself as the interpreter for your cells. Without the mechanical and chemical actions that *you* perform each time you eat—often without even thinking about it—your meal would not be translated into cell food that results in your health, healing, and energy.

From the physiological perspective, there are four phases of digestion—the cephalic phase, the esophageal phase, the gastric phase, and the intestinal phase. Each of those stages acts as a service station along the digestive superhighway. These service stations are integral to consider to calm your candida and restore your gut health.

Ready, Set, Go!

Digestion begins in a curious place . . . in your brain. The cephalic phase involves your brain and your central nervous system—the system in which your brain is located. *Cephalic* basically means "of or relating to the head." It's the sight, sound, smell, and thought of food that trigger the brain to transmit signals down your central nervous system through the biggest nerve in your body—the vagus nerve—and initiate both hunger and the digestive fires. (You can imagine this process in action by recalling walking into a kitchen that has bread or brownies baking in the oven, releasing an inviting smell that triggers your desire to eat.) *Vagus* literally means "wanderer," and this nerve does wander. It moves from the base of your brain down to your abdomen, and back again. It connects what is known as your gut-brain in your belly to your central brain in your head, creating what's known as your gut-brain axis.

The vagus nerve is responsible for actions such as hunger and elimination, gastric and enzyme release, gallbladder function, and intestinal blood flow. Yet while all those actions are related to your gastrointestinal function, your vagus nerve is part of your central nervous system, not your digestive system!

The term *gut-brain axis* is used to explain the two-way neural pathways between the emotional and cognitive centers of the brain (in your central nervous system) and your gut or enteric nervous system (which comprises the tissue that surrounds the organs in your digestive tract). A constant stream of electrical and chemical communication is moving between your gut and brain! This is why the physiological disturbances in your gut, such as candida overgrowth, can often be seen in mood, pain perception, and behavioral changes. The chemical communication mechanisms traveling between the two locations via your bloodstream include hormones, neurotransmitters, and immune messengers called cytokines, which can induce inflammation. Not only might your microflora affect your mood and memory, it will also manage your appetite and weaknesses for those munchies. An overgrowth of yeast will drive your cravings for sweets and sugars, possibly out of your control. This is because those yeasts lodged in your mucosal tissues thrive and survive on the sugars and starches that you consume as well as the more acidic environment that I have just described. Then, as also outlined, those sugars ferment and produce the gases and toxins that leave you feeling bloated, foggy, and fatigued. Reducing those refined starches and increasing your protein, as you will learn to do throughout the pages of this book, will go a long way in helping you gain back control of your gut-brain communications, as well as your life.

Before we leave the cephalic service station and the ways in which it both affects and is affected by your gut health, do consider that it's your brain that allows your body to move from the sympathetic phase of *fight and flight* to the parasympathetic phase of *rest and digest*. The parasympathetic nerves use more of those chemical messengers to take us into rest and digest, where we produce more saliva, enzymes, and acid that help move things along the digestive highway smoothly and efficiently. Without moving into rest and digest, guess what doesn't happen?

Chew on This

The next area to service your digestion is your mouth. While some of the initial steps involved in digestion are chemical, like those initiated in the brain, your mouth is the first location for mechanical digestion to occur. In your mouth, your mechanical digestion equals chewing. It seems simple enough, but it's an act we often rush through in favor of the swallow.

When you chew, your food breaks down and signals more hormones, enzymes, and gastric juices to initiate even more of those processes of digestion. The longer your food stays in this stage of dissolve—in this mechanical decomposition that occurs within your mouth, the more chemical directives are relayed and the easier digestion is on the rest of your body.

Well-chewed food glides easily through the esophagus and into the stomach. Dry and insufficiently chewed food has a more stilted journey through the entire digestive and metabolic chain reaction. Chewing alone can eliminate bloating, gas, and abdominal pain. Chewing is a cheap and easy way to increase the health and efficacy of your digestive system and benefit overall health. By freeing up the energy of the digestive system, imagine what else you might have the energy to accomplish!

Not only is your food dissected into smaller and smaller bits by your teeth when you chew, but the saliva in your mouth also produces enzymes that further disassemble your food's molecules into their successively smaller constituents. Saliva also contains softening agents to allow the food to be molded into a ball, called a bolus, for swallowing. In addition, you have more time to chemically alert the rest of your digestive system to start its engines.

The mouth is one of those opportune mucosal environments where candida can grow and thrive. This will typically only happen in those that are immune compromised, diabetic, very young, or very old. In babies we know candida overgrowth in the mouth as thrush, which appears as a white, curdled-looking substance on the tongue and on the sides of the mouth. This film is what you can imagine occurring in other mucosal areas of your body, such as your throat, your intestine, your urogenital tract, your anus, your respiratory tract, and even your skin. Several proteins produced in your saliva play a protective role in the oral cavity against candida overgrowth; under certain conditions, these proteins are prevented from doing their job.

Your Digestive Powerhouse

The next phase is the gastric phase; this service station is where the majority of digestion actually occurs—your stomach. Your stomach is responsible for the most effective breakdown of food particles and destruction of pathogens in your entire body. The stomach resembles a bagpipe in shape and it is situated between your rib cage, extending beneath the left ribs. It's connected to the mouth via the long tube called the esophagus (which comprises that esophageal phase of digestion) and is supported by a thick cluster of nerves, called the solar plexus.

When the stomach receives food, it secretes hydrochloric acid (HCL) to break down your individual macronutrients—specifically proteins—and kill most of the pathogens that might be in your food. It represents one of your digestive system's natural barriers, preventing the passage of opportunistic microorganisms into your intestines. The environment within the muscular walls of the stomach should be incredibly acidic. We're often mistakenly under the impression that we have too much stomach acid, yet the opposite is most often the case. Antacids only quell the symptoms of indigestion, yet they actually exacerbate the problem by depleting stomach acid that's already deficient.

As we age, the stomach is one of the first areas of the digestive system to decline in function, reducing its secretions and compromising its ability to both digest and utilize key nutrients from your diet—such as vitamin B_{12} and iron. Due to this diminishment of stomach acid production, the proper breakdown of your food is compromised and from there a number of health problems can ensue, including the bacterial or fungal overgrowth in the intestines that may have created the environment for your candida overgrowth to occur. Other symptoms of low stomach acid can include bad breath, belching, bloating, diarrhea, fatigue, food sensitivities, fullness immediately after eating, headaches, anemia or pernicious anemia, stomach pain immediately after eating or taking vitamins, and, of course, increased incidence of parasitic or yeast infections. Ouch! Clearly the stomach is a powerhouse with an impressive and influential job that needs to be done well. But, hey, many of those same signs and symptoms can be related to troubles farther down the digestive superhighway as well, indicating the intrinsic connections within your digestive system, from top to bottom.

Gimme Nutrients!

The small intestine is the organ that connects the stomach to the large intestine (the colon) and it's our next service station on your superhighway. Whereas the stomach takes the charge on digestion, or the breakdown of food, the small intestine governs absorption. This is the place where those microscopic nutrients traverse the barrier systems of the gut and move into your bloodstream to feed your cells.

The small intestine is located in the soft part of your belly, beneath your belly button, and is a 23-foot-long elastic and soft tube that's made of mucus, muscles, and membranes. It is coiled at your core and fits tightly contorted in your abdominal cavity. Go ahead and place your flat open hand on your belly in that area just beneath your belly button. This is the part of your body most in need of the service you will be delivering with your candida-free living and repair.

The small intestine converts food particles, separating the pure from the impure, into that fuel that feeds your cells. The proper functioning of the small intestine is critical for your nourishment. Practically all nutrient assimilation happens through fingerlike projections called villi that line the innards of the entire organ. Those villi are like a shag rug waving right inside your digestive tube. Approximately 90 percent of what you eat is assimilated by these villi.

Unfortunately, those little shags on the shag rug can get squashed when the intestines are damaged or inflamed. If this happens, you experience decreased nutrient uptake: you're in trouble and your digestive system is going to let you know it. The compression of those villi is what can happen in cases of celiac disease or nonceliac gluten sensitivity (NCGS). Those poor little shags get worn down. In fact, any condition that produces excess mucus in an irritated gut, will lead to the destruction of those minuscule yet vital villi. In addition to sensitivity to gluten, dairy and soy are other dietary factors that can contribute to what's called villous atrophy. Other inflammatory bowel conditions and parasitic infections can also destroy the proper function of the fingerlike projections. You now have an obvious state of intestinal inflammation, degeneration, and nutrient depletion—with the potential for further immune dysfunction.

The stage is now set for leaky gut and candida overgrowth to occur, two conditions that feed off each other's bearing on your health. The cells in your small intestine are designed to be extremely close to one another. This is what allows only the smallest of particles—those microscopic nutrients—to cross the intestinal barrier and move into your bloodstream. The slight space between those cells is called a tight gap junction. When the tight gap junctions become inflamed, they begin to expand and create more of a chasm between the cells, separating like bricks on an old building.

Portions of broken-down food molecules, too small for you to recognize as food but also too large for your cells to identify as fuel, leak through these fissures and into the bloodstream. The digestive environment is now one of intestinal permeability, a literal leaky gut, in consequence of which immune cells in the bloodstream are now called to chronic attention, battling fractured food molecules that are as foreign to them as any pathogenic invader. Your blood is trained to identify *fuel*, *self* (your other organs, glands, and tissues), and *other*. All of a sudden your dinner, even if it is one made with the very best intentions, clean and wholesome, is violating the rules of digestion and causing an immune system onslaught that over time dampens your resistance to infection and can even become so confused that it starts to strike self (otherwise known as an autoimmune attack).

As the inflammation in the intestines advances, provoked by the now-agitated climate, destruction of immune cells, located right within the walls of the intestine—where the majority of your immune cells reside—can become further compromised. With these surrounding conditions you are more susceptible to the overgrowth of opportunistic pathogens, such as candida. Then set in the signs and symptoms that make you feel sick—both inside your digestive system and out.

Signs and symptoms of leaky gut and candida differ from person to person, depending on the level of damage and the location of the afflicted tissues. It may be that you start to have myriad food sensitivities or nutritional deficiencies. You may experience diarrhea or constipation—or both! Erratic bowel patterns are a surefire sign of inflammation within the intestinal walls. When your white blood cells become confused by all they have to simultaneously contend with, compromised immunity will ensue, leaving you more prone to all sorts of sicknesses. Fatigue, memory loss, brain fog, depression, anxiety, and headache can be the result of toxin buildup moving through that gut-brain axis. The tissue in the brain barrier can be similar to that in the gut barrier and thus a leaky gut can lead to a leaky brain. Rashes, hives, breakouts, and eczema can indicate that your body is trying to release toxins through your biggest organ of detoxification, the skin. Both those nutrient deficiencies and the yeast overgrowth will cause unexplained hunger and cravings for sugar and starches and sometimes just more food in general, causing you to eat in excess, which further disrupts your digestive function and blood sugar regulation. Or, conversely, everything you eat leads to such abdominal discomfort that you're left hungry, malnourished, and confused about what will usher you out of this trap. All of these signs and symptoms ultimately point right back to the environment in your intestines, the microflora that is in need of rebalancing so that your gut can be reinstated as your number one barrier system from infection and disease.

Waste Station

The story doesn't end there. And by that I mean two things:

First, your digestive system doesn't end in your small intestine. The road continues. Ideally, as the food you eat travels along the superhighway of your digestive tract, the small intestine receives partially digested molecules from the stomach and processes them for further digestion by separating them into two categories: (1) what the body needs, which is assimilated into the bloodstream for circulation and delivery; and (2) waste, which is passed to the large intestine, for elimination—poop.

Those foreign substances that a healthy and not permeable gut is blocking from getting into the bloodstream can be chemical, bacterial, yeast, protozoa, and large molecules from food that we have eaten that have not been properly broken down or digested into their smallest particulates for assimilation into the bloodstream.

When these items are barred entry into the bloodstream, they move down the superhighway to your colon. The colon extracts the final bits of nutrients from the food, which include water as well as important minerals, such as calcium, magnesium, iron, zinc, and copper.

The combined health of the colon and presence of bowel bacteria (your colon is where most of the bacteria in your body resides) help you extract those lagging and important minerals from your food. When the colon stops functioning, absorption gets disrupted and these essential minerals, as well as many vitamins, may not be absorbed. And because it's part of this long, winding road from your mouth to your anus, the colon's health is affected by everything that's happening upstream. Any undigested food passed on from previous stages of ill digestion will linger in the colon and rot. The proteins putrefy, the carbohydrates ferment and create sugars to feed pathogenic bacterium and candida cultures, and the fats turn rancid and oxidize. In addition, an unhealthy colon is less able to expel through the feces the toxins that it accumulates, and, instead, it releases those toxins back into the bloodstream, where they, too, get absorbed.

As rotten food collects inside the colon, regular bowel movements can become compromised, get difficult, and sometimes, as you may know, are nonexistent.

Congestion of the colon can actually lead to the deformation of the organ. This includes loss of tone, swelling, decomposition, and general decline. This level of injury has a direct effect on your weight and energy as well as a referred association to everything from abdominal discomfort, back pain, sinus issues, headaches, and sore throats, to lethargy and fatigue. The end of our digestive superhighway is the rectum and anus, an area that can also be subject to inflammation and irritation from yeast overgrowth.

Testing for Candida and Getting a Proper Diagnosis

Now that you know some of the "how" and "why" of candida, you may be wondering how to get a proper candida diagnosis. Unfortunately, obtaining a diagnosis can be difficult. For starters, not all health or medical professionals know how to or believe in the value of testing for yeast. To complicate matters, not all testing methods are accurate. False negatives and positives can be the result of immune system imbalances.

When I suspect yeast overgrowth in a client, I like to start with a Yeast Assessment (see page 236). Completing this assessment allows you to consider your symptoms and gain a rating of the severity of those expressions in relation to potential yeast overgrowth.

What's Your Score? Date: _____   Score: _____

You'll hear more about this assessment later and how it pertains to the stages of the *Living Candida-Free* plan. Additionally, once you've taken the assessment, you may want to explore further testing to better understand what's present in your body. Certain tests will rate the severity of your yeast overgrowth. Do remember to continually come back to your assessment score. In my clinical opinion, if it walks like a duck and it talks like a duck, well . . . it's time to get unstuck.

Please keep in mind that diagnostic tests need to be administered through a healthcare professional. Unfortunately, finding a practitioner to partner with you to address your CRC isn't one-stop shopping. In certain medical arenas you may even find a candida diagnosis (and its related testing) to be considered bogus. It's important that you become the orchestrator of your own health care by seeking out a practitioner who understands your concerns and is willing to work with you to get to the roots of the cause and administer effective care. As you search for the appropriate support team, ask both yourself and the practitioner these key questions:

- If an MD, does she or he have holistic training?
- How many other patients with candida has she or he treated, and what is her or his success rate (i.e., how many had a full clearing of symptoms)?
- What is the practitioner's usual protocol? Does she or he combine antifungal pharmaceuticals with herbal or natural supplements?
- What kind of diet does she or he recommend?
- Which tests does she or he use? (See page 19 for my preferred tests.)

If you're pursuing an ND (licensed naturopathic physician) or nutritionist as your primary practitioner or for adjunct support, inquire about all of the above, as well as whether she or he has relationships with MDs who can prescribe antifungals if necessary.

One place to start is the Institute of Functional Medicine website (www.functional medicine.org). You can click on the "Find a Practitioner" tab or search for a naturopath, nutritionist, or well-trained integrative physician in your area (or you can find someone who works virtually as we do at Replenish PDX). As with any health professional, without further questions and research, you won't know about that person or practice's understanding of CRC.

Here are the diagnostic tests I find to be the most reliable for candida overgrowth:

- GI Effects Comprehensive Profile by Genova Diagnostics: This stool testing provides an expansive assessment of anaerobic gut microflora, evaluating bacteria, yeast, parasites, absorption, inflammation, and pharmaceutical and botanical agent sensitivities (meaning which antimicrobials agents will best work for your particular system).
- Metabolic Analysis Profile (Organic Acids) by Genova Diagnostics: This urinary assessment tests organic acids grouped according to their primary roles in metabolism.
- Anti-Candida Antibody Testing by Genova: This blood test looks at the immune response to candida, revealing the antibody reactivity to the yeast.

Note: Doctor's Data is another lab that provides similar tests to those listed here. Few other labs can accurately assess stool cultures or urine metabolites for these types of overgrowth.

A note for readers outside the United States: Although most of these tests aren't available in Canada, some larger centers will offer a few of them. If you seek a functional medicine specialist, such as a naturopath or holistic nutritionist, she or he will normally work with US-based labs to make use of the more specific tests. You can find international practitioners at the Institute of Functional Medicine website (www .functionalmedicine.org).

The End—and the Beginning

I said there were two reasons that the story doesn't end at your small intestine. Sure, the first reason is about your colon, which holds the serious task of ushering the adverse and extraneous out of your body. But the second reason is about hope.

I told you that I believe that you are not just what you eat, but what your body can *do* with what you eat. You can use the pages of this book to help you change what you eat. It's the first step, and it's essential to help you gain back command over the environment you likely didn't even know you were in charge of. Yet, you can't stop there. You can work with the information you'll find here to inform yourself as you take the first steps toward deep restoration and reparation—something you have likely been craving at the core, more than the sweet distractions.

By completing this chapter, you have made a tremendous step forward. You're now armed with the wisdom of "what's going on in there." You can now gain a little distance from your symptoms' cries and meet them with more understanding and compassion. You are now ready to hop into the driver's seat and drive on the superhighway of candida-free living. Congratulations!

Further Reading

DeLong, Leslie, and Nancy W. Burkhart. *General and Oral Pathology for the Dental Hygienist.* Philadelphia: Lippincott Williams & Wilkins, 2007.

Guarino, A., and E. M. M. Quigley, W. A. Walker, eds. *Probiotic Bacteria and Their Effect on Human Health and Well-Being.* Basel, NY: Karger, 2013.

Kamhi, Ellen, and Eugene R. Zampieron. *An Alternative Medicine Guide to Arthritis: Reverse Underlying Causes of Arthritis with Clinically Proven Alternative Therapies.* Berkeley: Celestial Arts, 2006.

CHAPTER 2

Cornerstones of the Anticandida Diet: Introducing the 4 D's

Receiving a diagnosis of "candida" can make you feel as if you've just embarked on the scariest, fastest roller coaster imaginable: it's that moment when you think, *Why did I put myself in this position?* As you inch toward the dizzying summit, the end may be in sight, but you suddenly realize you're not controlling the ride; and you just know there will be far too many peaks and plunges for your comfort level. But don't worry; there is a way to regain control and begin to enjoy the journey once again.

When your body struggles to control candida on its own, symptoms may worsen overnight. You wake up one morning with a raging sinus infection; or a raw, scarlet rash on your waistline; or oral thrush that is both painful and embarrassing. In reality, the candida has been stealthily growing over time, but it's easy to overlook the signs until it's so extreme that the excess manifests itself visibly, outside the body.

By the time readers find their way to my blog, they are often desperate for a cure. They're looking for something that can help them *today*, not a diet that will possibly require months before it shows any improvement. In fact, the most common question I see from readers is, "How long will it take to get better?" Another way of asking that same question is really, "How long will I be forced to follow this restrictive, punitive diet?"

To the first question, my answer is always, "I can't really say" (nor can anyone else; each person is unique, and the time it takes to heal and recover varies depending on the level of the candida overgrowth, the diet you've eaten in the past, your emotional and psychological state, your home environment, the city in which you live, and so on). However, I do believe that *everyone* can improve her or his condition and that almost everyone, if she or he adheres to an anticandida program, will eventually get better.

The second question is easier for me to answer because I think it's a bit of a red herring: *this diet does not need to feel restrictive*! When done right, an anticandida regimen includes lots of enticing, delectable foods even as it helps your body combat candida. (Oh, and in case there was any doubt, please note that you can't actually eat herring on this diet.)

I decided a few years ago that I will follow a maintenance form of an anticandida diet for the rest of my life. With that in mind, it's imperative that my diet include some foods that taste indulgent, foods that are bursting with flavor and that can be shared easily with others who may not have ever heard the word *candida*. Eating an anticandida diet doesn't have to feel like deprivation.

You may have read that the way to restore health on an anticandida diet is to "starve the yeast." But because *Candida albicans* is a normal part of a healthy digestive tract, it's virtually impossible to rid your body of every last vestige of candida. Consequently, I prefer to think of the approach as "putting the yeast on a diet"—in other words, a gentler process that will, in time, still diminish the overall load of candida enough to resolve the issue.

When I was impatient for my healing to progress more quickly, my ND used to remind me, "If you change the internal terrain, the yeast will eventually leave—there is no other possible outcome." In other words, creating an environment that's inhospitable or suboptimal for candida will eventually weaken it, and it will either die or move along. Stick with the anticandida program (diet, antifungals, supplements, and lifestyle changes) and, I firmly believe, you *will* get better—even if your initial condition is as severe as mine was.

As with many people who first begin an anticandida diet and assume their metabolism will reset itself in a couple of weeks, my early expectations were a tad unrealistic. I remember wondering, "How long will it take me to heal? How long before I can eat my beloved milk chocolate again, or glazed donuts?"

As the weeks progressed into months and I recognized improvements in how I felt, I turned to more realistic predictions. I scaled back my expectations and pondered instead, "How long before I can have bananas again? What about peanut butter?" It took decades of eating to excess, I reasoned, eating junk food, taking repeat courses of antibiotics, or ignoring the signals of my body before I reached my own profound level of illness, deteriorating a little bit at a time over the years until the result was entirely too evident and could no longer be ignored. Why would I expect to reverse all of that damage in just a month or even six weeks?

Dr. Ben Kim, chiropractor and author of a popular holistic health site, writes, "Please don't forget this fact: many chronic health challenges take years to develop, so it's unrealistic to expect such challenges to fully heal within months, even if you fully support your cleansing mechanisms."[1]

As you work through the early stages of the anticandida diet, it's essential to remember that healing isn't instantaneous. In our fast-paced, "this-morning's-trend-is-out-this-afternoon" world, we want instant gratification for just about everything. Your body will, hopefully, serve you well for many years to come. Think of this diet as building capital for the future, like paying mortgage on your dream home. It may require consistent payments over months—even years—to reach your ultimate goal. And sure, sometimes you might adjust the payments higher or lower; you could probably even skip a monthly payment once or twice over the life of the mortgage and still end up owning the home. But in general, the time and effort you put into the goal must be consistent over the long haul.

While the amount of time it takes is different for each person, I do believe that everyone is capable of healing with persistence and time. Give your body what it needs and it will correct the internal landscape.

My Anticandida Diet

Ask ten different candida experts what diet to follow to beat the condition, and you may just find yourself wondering: "Are they all talking about the same diet?" As it turns out, there are pretty much as many anticandida diets as there are people with CRC.

As we're learning with modern medicine in general, no one approach ever works equally well for everyone; there also exist multiple routes to the same result.

The hallmark of a good anticandida diet, in my opinion, is one that works *for you.* And while there are similarities among all the diets (they all want to kill off excessive yeast and prevent the yeast from proliferating), my own version is a compilation of what worked best for me over time, based on the many diets I've examined. Remember, what I offer is merely a guideline; you'll need to experiment to some extent to find what works best for you.

The diet I followed, like most anticandida diets, employed a four-pronged approach that, when taken together, is effective in getting candida under control so your body's own immune system can work to restore a healthy balance.

It's important to note that, while the four components work simultaneously to some extent, focusing on each one individually is essential to a successful anticandida protocol. Treating candida isn't like putting on a play, where one act follows the previous one in sequence; instead, you'll likely implement all four components at or around the same time, and their effects, and benefits, will overlap and work synergistically as you move through the program.

The "4 D's" Plan: Digestion, Detox, Dysbiosis, and Discord

The four cornerstones of the anticandida protocol are first, restoring good *digestion*; *detoxifying* the body; treating *dysbiosis* (repopulating the gut with healthful bacteria); and, finally, dealing with *discord* (psychological and emotional imbalances). Master these four components and you'll be well on your way to living "candida-free"!

Restoring Good Digestion: Gut Health

Embarking on a strict anticandida diet without also improving digestion is like trying to wash dishes with a tap that spouts muddy water; even when using the best soap available, unwanted dirt and grime will cling to the plates and bowls. The dishes will never be truly cleansed until the source of the water is sanitized and the tap runs clear.

When I was first diagnosed with IBS over twenty years ago, I suffered from constant bloating, gas, and what can only be described as debilitating constipation. After seeking help from a variety of doctors, I was finally referred to an acclaimed physician.

I was hopeful and expected some useful insights. Instead he recommended a powerful laxative, saying, "Use it once a week and clean yourself out. That will do it." He stopped short of flapping his hand and ending with, "Dismissed."

I'm embarrassed to say that I did attempt to follow his advice—once. I dutifully purchased the potion, drank it down, then promptly experienced shooting pains, nausea, and vomiting—all at the same time. I vowed never to take that heinous stuff again, and I haven't.

As is the case for so many people with candida, my digestive system was completely out of whack. True, you may be so accustomed to living with what is actually dysbiosis (an imbalance of the gut flora that affects digestion and overall health) and leaky gut that you no longer even register the slight bloating, or mild flatulence, or intermittent constipation, or irregular stools that occur on a far-too-regular basis. But candida thrives on your digestive upset and will continue to proliferate as long as digestion is compromised. So, it's imperative to support the breakdown of food while healing the intestinal lining at the same time. There are a few factors that play into this sequence.

The digestive tract, as you learned in Chapter 1, is really command central for your immune system and the starting point for myriad health issues, whether chronic diseases, such as arthritis, or systemic conditions, such as candida overgrowth. If digestion isn't working optimally, a whole host of other difficulties is likely to manifest at ostensibly unrelated parts of the body; and until digestion is repaired, your body won't flush toxins out effectively even if you do kill off all the excess candida with anticandida foods, supplements, or even prescription antifungals. With toxins lingering in the digestive tract, you may feel worse before you feel better.

But healing digestion can be an ongoing process, and one you want to initiate before you start to detox. There will, certainly, be some natural detoxification as soon as you begin consuming a cleaner diet, and that's totally normal. But most practitioners will suggest deferring any major attempts at detoxification until proper digestion has been restored, to avoid intense detox symptoms (also known as die-off; see page 35 for more on this).

In other words, if you are dealing with serious digestive issues in addition to candida, it makes sense to begin to treat those before you embark on the full anticandida diet protocol.

Get Digestion on Track: Eat to Heal Leaky Gut

As you know from Chapter 1, leaky gut is often concomitant with candida overgrowth. Healing leaky gut is crucial to your success with the diet, as it repairs the intestinal lining and prevents unwanted toxins or other organisms from entering the blood-stream, where they can wreak havoc on your immune and endocrine systems as well as on your mental health. Repairing digestion alone can often result in major improvements in symptoms.

The ACD is, by its nature, a diet that supports healing leaky gut. Eliminating gluten (very irritating to the digestive tract) and most sugars could prevent further damage. Eating nonallergenic foods and foods that heal and nourish the gut will also set you on the path toward wellness.

The following are gut-supportive foods that you'll want to consume on a regular basis:

Cabbage: Raw cabbage juice has been repeatedly shown to help heal ulcers and is very soothing to the entire digestive tract. Just eating cabbage on a daily, or almost daily, basis can be beneficial to digestion as well.[2]

According to Phyllis A. Balch in *Prescription for Dietary Wellness*, "The high levels of vitamin A aid in tissue rejuvenation, and the sulfur content helps fight infection and protects the skin from eczema and other rashes. In its raw form and especially as a juice, cabbage contains ascorbigen, formerly called cabbagen or vitamin U, which heals and protects against stomach ulcers."[3] And let's not forget that it tastes good, too! (Note: Under certain conditions, raw cabbage can cause further digestive distress. If you find this to be true when you eat cabbage, try it cooked or in its fermented form— lacto-fermented sauerkraut—or stick with the juice; or begin with small quantities to see how you feel.)

Soaked or sprouted nuts, seeds, gluten-free grains, and legumes: Sprouts are one of the healthiest foods you can eat. Think about sprouts in relation to tending a garden: after you plant and water a seed, tender sprouts emerge from the germinating seeds; these grow into full plants. In the case of nuts, grains, and legumes, these might be the "seeds" for an almond tree, a paddy of rice grass, or a bean pod. It's the sprout that develops, like a plant embryo, supplying nourishment to the growing plant and allowing it to flourish. It makes sense that sprouts would be filled with all kinds of nutrients, more so than the dry nut, seed, or legume.

In addition to their supernutrient qualities, sprouts are generally more easily digested than are the unsprouted or unsoaked forms of the same food. Nuts and seeds contain compounds to protect them from damage until they are ready to germinate; the two most common are called phytates and enzyme inhibitors. These protect the seed but make digestion more difficult for humans. Phytic acid binds to minerals (magnesium, zinc, calcium, and others), thereby inhibiting digestion. Soaking nuts and seeds helps reduce the phytates and also acts as a catalyst to increase enzymes in food, which also improves digestibility.[4] In addition, soaked nuts and seeds have a softer texture and taste sweeter than their dry counterparts. If you miss crunchy nuts, the soaked nuts can be dehydrated or dried in the oven (see page 97).

Grains, whether they are gluten-free or not, also contain phytates as well as substances called lectins that interfere with proper digestion. Soaking the grains before cooking helps reduce these compounds as well.[5]

In other words, it makes sense to first soak nuts, seeds, and grains before cooking and/or eating them, and to either soak or sprout legumes. And although it's not always practical or possible, it's a great practice to implement as often as you can, especially in the early stages of the diet. For how-tos, see Chapter 6.

Cultured foods: Cultured (a.k.a. lacto-fermented) foods, such as homemade sauerkraut, kimchi (Korean spicy sauerkraut), and beet kvass are naturally fermented. These foods contain innate probiotics that can aid in intestinal repair and also help repopulate the gut with "good" bacteria. Naturally fermented foods also contain more concentrated, and a more diverse variety of, bacteria than can usually be provided by a supplement alone.[6] Given that our guts contain more bacterial cells than the number of cells in our whole body, it's imperative that we keep those numbers up!

Start by eating 1 tablespoon (15 ml) of cultured veggies a day at the beginning of the diet, then increase to about ¼ cup (60 ml) per day over time. These days, I consume a tablespoon or two (15 to 30 ml) almost every day. I love to eat them in wraps, in my "Toronto" Sandwich (page 151), or just as a quick snack. I've come to love salads tossed with sauerkraut, too (as in the Fennel, Brussels Sprout, and Edamame Salad, page 166).

It's easy to make cultured vegetables at home, and, after the initial work of setting up the jars, you can basically forget about them until they're ready (see page 109 for how-tos).

Omega-3 oils: Omega-3 oils are anti-inflammatory and also help heal the gut lining. Most people know that omega-3s are available through fish oil, but they are also found in chia seeds, flaxseeds, walnuts, and some algae (which is where the fish get their own omega-3s!).[7]

Coconut oil: Unlike other saturated fats, coconut oil is a medium-chain fatty acid that's digested more readily and easily. It also contains antifungal properties that combat candida while nourishing your intestinal lining (for more on coconut oil, see page 45).

Get Digestion on Track: Clean Up Your Food!

A second way to help improve digestion is to avoid poor-quality food, processed food, or food that contains artificial or toxic substances; these can all contribute to leaky gut and compromised digestion. Aim to avoid these toxins by eating good, clean, whole foods. Remember, each time you choose what to eat, you support either speeding up or slowing down your recovery process.

NAG Yourself

Eat foods free of additives, artificial colorings, artificial flavorings, or other chemicals.

When I was in nutrition school, we were taught that an ideal diet is represented by the acronym NAG, which stands for "natural, alive, good quality." I've stuck with NAG principles for my own diet since then, and it applies perfectly to the ACD as well.

For our purposes here, I define *natural* as the opposite of *processed*. This means foods that are as close as possible to their original state, the way they came out of the ground (or off the animal). If a food has been processed, it should be avoided as much as possible.

For example, anything you do to change the original form of a food is, technically, processing it. On the other hand, some types of processing, especially if they can be reproduced easily at home, are preferable to others.

I would never use jam made in a factory with sugar, pectin, or artificial colors. However, when I cook up my own blueberry jam with organic blueberries, a bit of filtered water, and stevia, I'm fine with that even though it's technically "processed." Similarly, while my preference whenever possible is to use whole, fresh ingredients, sometimes life requires shortcuts.

My aim here is to ensure that the shortcuts don't interfere with healing. So, before you choose prepared or packaged foods, consider what's been changed, how much has been added, and how it's been "processed."

For instance, dried organic beans that have been soaked at home in filtered water, drained, then cooked, would be the first choice and most natural option for beans. However, I will sometimes grab a (non-BPA) can of organic chickpeas, say, rinse it very (very!) well to remove excess sodium, and use those chickpeas in My Favorite Hummus (page 161) or Quick and Easy Chard and Chickpea Soup (page 149). This is a fine alternative if you're pressed for time, can't find fresh, or feel too exhausted to prepare the fresh alternative all the time; just try to keep those "shortcut" incidents to a minimum for best results.

By *alive*, I mean raw foods—those that contain live enzymes. Raw foods are a part of the Candida-Free plan.

Raw Foods Are Superclean

Raw foods are a great choice for an anticandida diet. They contain natural enzymes that aid in digestion as well as maximum levels of nutrients that your body needs (the exceptions are a few foods with nutrients more easily absorbable when cooked—spinach, tomatoes, and a few others). It's a good idea to provide your body with as many fresh, raw ingredients as you can every day.

My rule of thumb is to consume 50 percent or more raw food at every meal if possible, and focus particularly on dark leafy greens, the stars of the vegetable kingdom. You can enjoy them in smoothies, salads, wraps, or any other way you think of! Juicing is a particularly good means to enjoy the benefits of raw vegetables. See the recipe chapters in Part 2 for ideas.

Go for Good-Quality and Organic

One of the easiest ways to clean up your diet is to buy organic ingredients as much as possible. Certified organic foods are grown and harvested without the use of synthetic chemical pesticides or fertilizers; and they are, by definition, free of genetically modified organisms (GMOs), though in recent years there have been reports of some cross-contamination of GMO seeds with organic crops.[8]

While there have been conflicting reports about whether organic produce contains more vitamins and minerals than conventionally grown foods, a recent meta study in July 2014 found that organic food does, indeed, provide more nutrients, and retains fewer pesticide residues, than do conventionally grown foods.[9]

It's also worth noting that some studies have found genetically modified foods to cause changes in the intestinal tract and digestive organs (liver, pancreas, kidneys, and more),[10] as well as in immune system function. And because GMOs aren't currently (at the time of this writing) labeled, unless we eat organic, we might inadvertently be consuming genetically modified organisms that contribute to our digestive woes—thereby increasing our difficulties with candida as well.

But organic is expensive, and very few of us can afford to eat entirely organic menus (I certainly can't). In reality, even Bill Gates likely couldn't eat 100 percent organic food if he decided to do so, because many foods aren't available in organic varieties at all locations.

So, what's the best approach? Here are my personal "rules" when it comes to organic food.

Nonnegotiable Foods

The Dirty Dozen: I rely on the annually updated Environmental Working Group's dual list of a Dirty Dozen and Clean Fifteen.[11] These lists, respectively, name the twelve fruits and vegetables that contain the largest pesticide residues and the fifteen with the least pesticide residues for that year. In other words, I ensure that if I consume any produce listed among the Dirty Dozen, it is organic as much as is possible. I avoid buying certain foods (e.g., strawberries) even if they're in season, if I can't find organic ones. Similarly, if you shop at a farmers' market for your produce, it's easy to get to know your local farmers and you can find out whether they use pesticides on their crops, even if they're not certified organic. Another option, of course, is to grow your own, without the use of chemicals.

Another trick to use if you don't have the EWG list on hand (or memorized) is to consider whether the portion of the fruit or vegetable you wish to eat is protected by a peel you can remove. Avocados, for instance, are shielded by a thick, inedible skin; whereas strawberries or raspberries have porous skins and crevices in which sprayed chemical residues can hide, even after washing.

On the other hand, I'm okay eating nonorganic when it's among the Clean Fifteen, or if it's impossible to get fresh organic options outside the Dirty Dozen. In my opinion, it's better to consume lots of fresh produce than none at all, even if the produce is not organic (be sure to clean well and peel if possible). And don't forget that many of these foods are available in organic form in the freezer section of your supermarket or local health food store.

Animal products: There are many problems associated with eating animal products, especially when you're trying to detoxify and clean up your body. If you've ever been on a detox diet or cleanse, you likely recall that it doesn't contain a lot of pork loin or lobster. In fact, some of the worst offenders, when it comes to foods that contain chemicals, drugs, hormones, and other nasty compounds, are meats, shellfish, eggs, and dairy products.

If you are serious about clearing up your candida and you still wish to eat animal products, you'll need to buy organic. Having a little dose of erythromycin or anabolic steroids[12] along with your hamburger just isn't conducive to clearing out the yeast. In addition, it's important to explore how the animals were raised and the feed they were provided as well (even organic farmers sometimes give their cows corn, a food the animals would never consume in nature).

Foods That Cause Negative Reactions

It's a sad fact of twenty-first-century life that most of us these days either know some-one with a serious allergy, or have heard stories about deathly allergies. But "true" aller-gies are still fairly rare, with only between 4 and 5 percent of the population suffering from them.[13] Most people who have true allergies are aware of them: there is an imme-diate, classic allergic reaction causing difficulty breathing, hives, swelling, and so on.

Many more of us, however, are victim to delayed reactions or sensitivities, partly connected to leaky gut or poor digestion. This type of reaction can occur anywhere from thirty minutes to days after we ingest the offending foods. Common culprits include wheat, gluten, dairy, soy, corn, and food additives or preservatives.

It only makes sense to avoid foods that cause you digestive distress, discomfort, itching, sinus congestion, inflammation, or any other negative reactions, whether or not you've been diagnosed as "allergic." In these cases, your symptoms are an indica-tion that the food triggers an alarm reaction in the immune system. And since the immune system of anyone with CRC is already likely overburdened, reducing any strain possible on the system will allow the body to deal more effectively with excess candida. That's also why the diet eliminates foods that are most likely to set off aller-gies or sensitivities.

Easily Digested Foods

Fried foods, as well as certain other "heavy" foods, tend to be more difficult to di-gest. Of the three macronutrients, fat (as opposed to protein and carbohydrates) takes longest for the digestive system to break down into fatty acids that can be used by the cells in your body. For many of us, consuming too much fat generates a feeling of heaviness, like a weight inside the stomach. Ideally, you want your food to be broken down efficiently and make its way through the digestive tract without overtaxing the entire system, so as to obtain the fuel and energy it needs from the food you consume.

Right now, it's important to support healthy digestion, making the process as easy and efficient as it can be. Consequently, reducing foods with heavy fat concentrations is a good idea. At the same time, we know that the fat in food both improves taste and allows us to feel sated so we don't run off on a cookie bender at 9:47 p.m. In other words, focus on healthy fats (see "healthy oils" on page 43) and be sure you don't eliminate them completely.

Get Digestion on Track: Start the Juices Flowing

One key tactic to improve digestion is optimizing proper secretions (e.g., digestive enzymes or hydrochloric acid in the stomach) to break down food effectively.

What we think of as "digestive juices" actually begins in the mouth with the first bite of any food, when saliva mingles with starch in foods to begin to break them down. As you read in Chapter 1, ensuring that food is mixed with appropriate digestive enzymes at each stage of the digestive tract, as well as with sufficient hydrochloric acid in the stomach, is essential for good digestion. In addition, as we age, the amount of hydrochloric acid our bodies produce naturally decreases, and digestion isn't always as efficient as it had been. Here are a few tricks you can employ to jump-start proper digestion, even before you begin to eat.

Got lemons? Make lemonade. About twenty minutes before you eat breakfast (you *are* eating breakfast, right?), start the day with a glass of pure, room-temperature or slightly warm water with the juice of one-half lemon squeezed into it.

Although lemon juice is acidic, it is highly alkalizing once in the body, and it stimulates the stomach to begin producing some of its natural digestive juices. It's a very gentle means to get things going before you eat in the morning, and it also helps promote healthy liver functioning. Note: Be careful with fresh lemon water, though, as it can affect the enamel of your teeth! Either rinse with clear water right after drinking (don't brush your teeth; that just scrubs your teeth with the acids in the lemon juice); or use a straw to drink your lemon water.

Sip on raw apple cider vinegar. Raw apple cider vinegar can be added to water or beverages for a similar effect to lemon juice on digestion. Further, the raw form (look for vinegar with the cloudy "mother" still in it) is a naturally fermented food that may be alkalizing and provide probiotic benefits as well. Start with about 1 teaspoon (5 ml) in room-temperature water and work up to 1 tablespoon (15 ml). I use it often, in my ACD-Friendly Fruity Sipper (page 116).

Relax—and digest. A relaxed mind and body when you eat allow your digestive system to do its work to properly break down food. When you're tense or too stressed, blood is directed away from the stomach and your food doesn't receive the digestive attention it deserves. The result is often bloating or other uncomfortable symptoms later on.

One trick to prompt a relaxation response is to close your eyes and take three deep breaths into your belly right before you begin to eat. The long, slow breaths will trigger the parasympathetic nervous system, in charge of relaxing the muscles, and will also put you in the right mind-set to best appreciate and enjoy your food. Saying grace accomplishes this same goal of stopping to reflect and relax before eating. So often, traditional approaches hit the right note, even if the people who created them had different motivations!

Get on the "chew-chew" train. Holistic nutritionists have a saying: "Drink your food and chew your liquids." In other words, the more you chew your food (as close to the "drinkable" liquid state as possible), the more it combines with salivary digestive enzymes, beginning the process of properly breaking down the food. Similarly, we forget that smoothies and juices are made from whole foods that must also be mixed with digestive enzymes to break down completely. By "chewing" your drinks (swishing them around a bit in your mouth so that you produce some saliva to mix with them), you ensure better digestion of these nutritional powerhouses, too.

Wait for water (and serve it at room temperature). Too much water during meals can interfere with digestion by diluting the natural digestive juices; and cold water interferes even more. It's best to wait a while after you've eaten to drink water, but, if you do imbibe with your meals, ensure that it's room temperature, and sip rather than slurp. But do be sure to remain hydrated throughout the diet, as this will help to support the body and flush out toxins. Most people should drink a minimum of six to eight glasses of room-temperature, filtered water throughout the day between meals.

Detoxifying Your Body and Environment

Our bodies are designed for ongoing detoxification, which happens naturally every day through the internal filters (liver and kidneys) as well as our skin (via sweating) and digestive tract (via elimination). In general, each person's toxicity is based on the amount of toxins to which she or he is exposed, along with the health and efficiency of the detox organs. Given the postindustrial, pollutant-filled, and toxin-heavy world we live in, however, it's my belief that almost everyone's body today deals with an excessive toxic load.

In addition, people with CRC are even more likely to harbor an overload of toxins, as their normal channels for detoxification are working suboptimally. As excessive yeast is eliminated through diet or the use of antifungal supplements or prescription medications, supporting the detoxification process will help increase and enhance healing by removing some of the other antipathetic organisms (e.g., germs, bacteria, or parasites), chemicals, and metals from the body.

Once you've improved digestive function and your gut is better able to handle detoxification, your practitioner may decide to implement some additional detoxing.

Some of the most common methods to hasten or increase detoxification include saunas (particularly infrared saunas), colonics,[14] chelation (for heavy metal detox), consuming herbs and supplements (see page 37), dry brushing (a practice of using a natural-bristle brush to stimulate the lymph pathways each day before showering), or using a rebounder (mini-trampoline) for a few minutes a day to increase the flow of lymph in the body.

Finally, one of the best ways to detox your body each day is through sleep. Honoring the circadian rhythm and getting to bed by 10 p.m. will give your body the rest it needs to function optimally. See Chapter 14 for more ideas on detoxing your self-care products, cleansers, and home.

It's also important while detoxing to support the body's own detoxification systems, particularly the filters (liver and kidney), which will be working overtime during this period. For this reason, I also include supplements and herbs for liver and kidney support in the list of supplements (see pages 58–61). And, of course, don't forget to drink lots of water to help flush away those toxins via the urinary system!

The Herxheimer Reaction

As you learned in Chapter 1, when the yeast begins to die off in large numbers, it releases mycotoxins, such as alcohol or acetaldehyde, into the system that can actually make you feel worse before you feel better. This phenomenon is known as a healing crisis, or Jarisch-Herxheimer reaction.[15] Ironically, even though you may feel worse for a short while, this reaction actually indicates that the program is working because the yeast must die off to trigger it.

Symptoms usually resolve within a week, but, in general, they signal that your own detoxification pathways aren't able to handle the increased toxic load. And if symptoms are intense or continue, always check with your health-care provider before continuing with the diet!

Typical die-off symptoms are flulike (low fever, muscle aches, headache, flushing, muscle pain), nausea, inflammation, or appearance/return of skin rashes or yeast infections (vaginal or oral thrush).

Treating Dysbiosis: Repopulate the Good Bacteria in the Gut

The internal terrain of the digestive tract, as you learned in Chapter 1, is normally populated with a large variety of microorganisms, from bacteria to fungi and parasites. When the normal intestinal flora is healthy, these toxins are kept in check and pose no threat to your health. When you're diagnosed with candida-related complex, however, it means your digestive tract's intestinal flora is out of balance and the "good" bacteria have been replaced to some extent with "bad" organisms; this is known as dysbiosis. As you eliminate excess candida, it's also essential to "reinoculate," or repopulate the intestines with the good guys once again.

While we haven't identified every single probiotic that normally exists in the digestive tract (there are far too many!), we do know that probiotics are essential for a healthy gut and that they perform key tasks related to immune function and proper digestion. The most common strains of probiotics in the body are *Lactobacillus acidophilus, Bifidobacteria bifidum*, and *Eschericia coli*,[16] so these are the strains you will find most in supplements. While supplements are extremely helpful, they may not, however, be the most effective means to restore necessary beneficial bacteria; recent research suggests that consuming lacto-fermented (naturally fermented) foods is also a key step.

According to Dr. Natasha Campbell-McBride, founder of the GAPS (Gut and Psychology Syndrome) diet, naturally fermented foods can contain up to one hundred times the amount of probiotics found in a good supplement, and they also offer a wider variety of probiotic strains.[17] In her book *The Body Ecology Diet*, Donna Gates also writes extensively about the importance of naturally fermented foods in reestablishing healthy gut bacteria.[18] In the previous section I spoke about exactly which foods to consume to heal leaky gut. These should be eaten in conjunction with any probiotic supplements. Some diets suggest waiting until much of the candida has died off before starting to take probiotics; I believe that they are useful throughout the process, and that a generous amount of these good bacteria in the system throughout the process allows for faster repopulation of gut bacteria as the candida dies off.

For more on supplements, see page 58.

Dealing with Psychological and Emotional Discord

It almost goes without saying that someone living with candida also faces an inordinate amount of stress. The condition alone, with its debilitating symptoms and fuzzy thinking, is enough to generate anxiety.

Having dealt with candida for as long as I have and having undergone myriad treatments for the condition, I've come to believe that stress is perhaps one of the *most* critical factors to address so as to ensure recovery. You may very well do everything "right," as I did, over a period of time, but, if you still don't see results, I'd suggest finding ways to combat excessive stress (even what Hans Selye dubbed "eustress," or "good" stress, can depress immune function, so stress management is always a good idea whether or not you feel the effects consciously).

Suggestions to Manage Stress

Each person deals with stress differently, of course, but here are some tried-and-true methods. (Note that neither chemical nor prescription therapy for stress or anxiety appear here.)

Meditation: This is probably the single most effective method for reducing stress and improving one's psychological ability to deal with it; yoga provides some of these same benefits, too. As Jon Kabat-Zinn outlines in his seminal book, *Full Catastrophe Living*,[19] our attitudes, states of mind, and beliefs can all affect our health; likewise, health can be improved through mindfulness meditation. Many other studies have confirmed that meditation improves one's health by reducing stress and boosting immune function—both of which will help immensely to combat your candida.[20]

Talk therapy—professional or otherwise: Talking with a compassionate and concerned friend, relative, clergy member, therapist, or other trusted professional can help reduce stress. Studies have shown that people with social support, either through individuals, friends, groups, or the community, are better able to deal with life's stressors and remain healthier than those with poor social support.[21]

Natural Herbs and Supplements: As with prescription drugs, there are a variety of herbs, herbal teas, supplements, or homeopathic remedies designed to help reduce stress. Speak with your health-care practitioner if you're interested in trying some of these.

Animals: Most of us have heard that petting a dog or cat can lower blood pressure and reduce stress. In fact, interacting with your pet lowers cortisol (stress hormone) levels and increases serotonin ("feel good" chemicals) in the body. This seems to work regardless of the pet—even watching fish swim can have a beneficial effect on you. If you have a pet, take advantage of this extra benefit it offers.[22]

Nature: For many people, a walk or other activity in nature is a natural stress reducer. A walk along the beach, a hike in the woods, biking on a trail, even jogging through the neighborhood can all help alleviate stress.

Hobbies and personal interests: The act of being fully engaged in an enjoyable activity that requires complete mastery and complete mental focus is not only satisfying to most of us; it also precludes negative emotions like anxiety or worry.[23] In this way, becoming involved in fulfilling hobbies can also help alleviate stress by otherwise occupying the mind. Besides, hobbies are just fun.

Change your perception of stress: Kelly McGonigal (a professor of psychology at Stanford University's School of Medicine and author of *The Willpower Instinct*) suggests that our attitude toward stress may influence the physical outcome more than the stress itself. In other words, perceiving stress as something that may, ultimately, allow your body to rise to the challenge at hand can work to improve your health in the long run even if the original stressor remains.[24]

Exercise: For many people, a turn on the treadmill, lifting weights, aerobics classes, or other indoor fitness activities are a fine alternative to outdoor activities that can also reduce overall stress levels.

CHAPTER 3

Rebalancing Your Body Through Food and Lifestyle: The ACD Plan

If you've read or researched anything about candida, you've likely encountered a plethora of different diets, many of which have already achieved a certain level of fame and influence. Some of these allow almost all nuts and seeds; some prohibit grains while others allow gluten-free grains, or even some non-gluten-free ones (e.g., spelt and barley); some permit legumes while others remove them entirely.

I've also seen several approaches that advocate "eradicating" and "starving" the candida, with the caveat that even a mild slipup would hurtle you back to the very first day of the diet. I see a twofold problem with this mind-set: first, you can never completely "starve" the candida (nor would you want to) because it's impossible to rid your system of the organism entirely (and some is actually necessary). At best, an anticandida diet diminishes the yeast population sufficiently that the body's own immune system takes over to achieve homeostasis once again. So, to my mind, the ACD is more like "putting candida on a diet" so it will gradually slim down until it reaches a manageable population, one that works symbiotically in your body as it is meant to do.

Second, while I suggest *never* consciously breaking the diet, sometimes life intervenes. If it turns out that you consume something off-target and realize it later, my suggestion is to simply continue from that point onward and pick up where you left off. If you experience slipups along the way but maintain the diet overall, your progress may be slower and your healing may take longer, but eventually, you'll still heal. In fact, given my own progress through the diet, I'd say that second scenario is the one I fell into.

As a result, I offer an anticandida regimen that provides the maximum number of options while still targeting excess yeast in the body. As I've mentioned before, everyone is different. I had a very extreme case; your health may require a less stringent plan. Regardless of where you begin, once your system has adjusted to a yeast-free diet, I also provide a slightly stricter version that can speed up the process if you wish. I call this the "Fast Track" (see page 48 for more details).

Whichever version you choose, it's important to remember the Four D's that underpin the diet. As you begin to eliminate excess candida by consuming healthful, anticandida foods and (in most cases) taking anticandida supplements or prescription antifungals, you'll undoubtedly improve digestion, experience some detox symptoms, treat dysbiosis to repopulate the good gut bacteria, and, ideally, tackle any psychological discord that may linger for you as well; all of the Four D's should coexist as you make your way through the stages of the diet.

Eat to Beat Candida: Overview of the ACD Plan

Depending on your personal genome, your physical and psychological history, your present environment, your medical history, and the severity of candida overgrowth in your system, your own diet will vary to a lesser or greater extent from what other people require. Moreover, what doesn't work at the very beginning may be fine later on.

I will explain the reasoning behind my choices, but please, if anything here doesn't work for you or doesn't feel right, by all means, don't use it. As I am not a doctor or medical professional, I can't recommend what you should or shouldn't do. You should never start this or any diet without first consulting your own physician or qualified health-care practitioner. Work with her or him to determine which of the following recommendations fits well within your own body and lifestyle.

While the amount of time it takes is different for every person, I do believe that everyone is capable of healing, with persistence and time. Give your body what it needs and it *will* correct the internal landscape eventually.

As I mentioned earlier, a successful anticandida diet works on various levels concurrently: repairing digestion, detoxifying, correcting dysbiosis, all while attending to any emotional or psychological discord. Most people will experience some degree of die-off, or Herxheimer reaction (see page 35).

To help mitigate the die-off period, this diet is designed with the fewest ingredient restrictions possible while still maintaining a regime that will help your body fight off excess candida. However, if you find that your own detox reaction is minimal, you may decide to shift to the more challenging "Fast Track" version of the diet after the first two weeks to speed up your progress. (Note that everyone should start with *at least* two weeks on the basic diet described on pages 41–47, however.)

I've found that the best way to approach this program is through an ongoing process in which you reassess your situation every three months or so, and then revise your diet accordingly. In other words, once you begin the ACD, you should always return to the Yeast Assessment form (see page 236) after each three-month period to track your progress and determine whether to move on to a successive stage of the diet.

Before You Begin: Assess Your Symptoms

Once you've filled out the Yeast Assessment form (see page 236), you'll have a good idea of how severe your symptoms are. Your score will also give you a baseline for later assessments down the road. If you haven't yet, go ahead and do the assessment and come back here to read about getting started on the diet.

Your Basic Anticandida Diet

This is the diet you should follow when you start your anticandida program.

The foods in this list all serve to nourish your body well, help heal the gut, and support detoxification as you work through the stages of the diet. This is the diet that I ate throughout my first six months or so on the program. (Note that some of these ingredients or foods may be unfamiliar; you'll learn more about them a bit later in this chapter and in Chapter 5.)

Foods to Eat Freely
- All vegetables except mushrooms and potatoes (exceptions: red-skinned potatoes are fine in moderation; medicinal mushrooms, such as shiitake or reishi, are okay if used sparingly)
- Sprouts made from seeds, vegetables, or legumes, except mung bean sprouts
- Fruits: only lemon, lime, fresh or frozen unsweetened cranberries, avocado
- All fresh raw nuts and seeds (okay to toast them yourself) *except those below*

YOUR ACD PLAN: OVERVIEW

Assess Your Symptoms → Stage 1

Work in consultation with your practitioner to determine which supplements and/or prescription antifungals you should take.

After 2 weeks on Stage 1 → either continue with diet *or* move to Fast Track

Work in consultation with your practitioner to determine which supplements and/or prescription antifungals you should take.

After 2–3 months: reassess and move to Stage 2, if appropriate.

Work in consultation with your practitioner to determine which supplements and/or prescription antifungals you should take, and which you can reduce or eliminate at this point.

After 2–3 months: reassess and move to Stage 3, if appropriate.

Work in consultation with your practitioner to determine which supplements and/or prescription antifungals you should take, and which you can begin to reduce or eliminate at this point.

After 6 months: remain at Stage 3 or add selected foods, if appropriate

Work in consultation with your practitioner to determine which supplements and/or prescription antifungals you should take, and which you can begin to reduce or eliminate at this point.

For further details on each stage, see page 40.

- Gluten-free grains and pseudo-grains: brown rice (any variety), millet, buckwheat, quinoa, amaranth. No more than one serving per day.
- Lacto-fermented sauerkraut, kimchi, or homemade cultured vegetables (if store-bought, must be the kind that contain live bacteria and have to be refrigerated; no commercial pickles, sauerkraut, etc.)
- Beans and legumes except split peas (may include soy as listed below; no tofu or soy milk)

- Tempeh, miso, wheat-free tamari, or Bragg Liquid Aminos; coconut aminos
- Beverages: herbal teas; green tea, including matcha (but not jasmine); filtered water; homemade nut and/or seed milks
- Juices: freshly juiced green juices (without fruit added); unsweetened 100 percent cranberry juice; and wheatgrass juice, if tolerated
- Sea veggies: nori, arame, wakame, etc.
- Algae: spirulina, chlorella, etc.
- Black olives cured in oil (the ones I can get are called infornata)
- Healthy oils: organic coconut, olive, sesame
- Other (usually small amounts as part of some other recipe): carob powder, psyllium seed husk, tiny amounts of baking powder or xanthan gum, herbs and spices, vanilla powder, protein powder (hemp or pea/bean protein are best)

In addition, see the list of the ACD Superstar foods (see page 40), for particularly helpful choices.

A Note to Omnivores

While this is a vegan program and I recommend vegan food if you follow it, I realize that some people are not vegans. If you choose, you can add these "Andrea-approved" animal proteins to any of the main dishes in the recipe section.

- Wild fish
- Grass-fed, pastured, and wild meats
- Pastured poultry and game
- Bone and meat broths

Please note, however, that the following restrictions apply even if you normally eat these foods: conventional red meat, tuna, farmed salmon, shellfish (shrimp, crab legs, lobster, etc.), eggs, dairy (cheese, milk, butter, yogurt, etc.), prepared or deli meats (cold cuts, bacon, hot dogs, sausages, etc.).

Foods to Avoid

Don't consume any of the following while on the program:

- Alcohol or items with any alcohol in the ingredients

- Any sweeteners of any kind, whether natural or artificial, except stevia, yacon, or lo han guo
- Caffeine, including coffee, caffeinated soft drinks, teas, and cocoa/hot chocolate (exceptions: green teas and raw cacao powder)
- Grain-based coffee substitutes (Dandy Blend is allowed later on; use it if you're desperate!)
- Grains not listed under "Foods to Eat Freely": rolled oats (including gluten-free oats), wheat, kamut, spelt, barley, triticale, corn, rye, white rice
- Yeast or anything containing yeast, including nutritional yeast
- Starches, such as tapioca starch, cornstarch, arrowroot, potato starch
- Packaged cereals and puffed grains (e.g., rice cakes)
- Prepared baked goods of any kind (bread, cookies, cakes, pastries, crackers, muffins, brownies, bars, waffles, etc.)
- Prepared (or homemade) goods that contain even a *smidge* of restricted grains or starches
- Potatoes (exception: red-skinned, which are okay); mushrooms (exception: some medicinal ones are okay)
- Dried fruits and/or vegetables (e.g., no sun-dried tomatoes or raisins)
- Marinated foods (e.g., premarinated artichoke hearts; most olives)
- Canned, jarred, prepackaged or premixed foods unless they contain only one or two whole food ingredients that are easily identified (e.g., canned tomatoes, canned artichoke hearts, canned beans)
- Prepared condiments, such as ketchup, mustard, relish, jam, jelly, peanut butter
- Prepared salad dressings or mayonnaise
- Prepared sauces (Tabasco, Worcestershire, black bean, Asian fish sauce, etc.)
- Peanuts or pistachios

Anticandida Superstar Foods

As you'll see when you browse through the recipe section and sample meal plans, it's really not difficult to prepare complete, delicious meals from these ingredients! And while all of the "Foods to Eat Freely" list is open to you at any time, you can support the

HOW CAN I TELL WHETHER I CAN TOLERATE CERTAIN FOODS?

As Andrea noted in Chapter 1, it's sometimes hard to understand why your roommate or spouse or best friend can eat a hot fudge sundae without experiencing the same fatigue, brain fog, and bloating that might befall you. And it doesn't seem fair! But what about seemingly healthy foods, such as chia seeds or parsnip? Because candida can affect each one of us differently, it's complicated.

For example, if you introduce cauliflower and then notice an increase in your symptoms (or a return of previously cleared symptoms) within a day or two, cauliflower might not work for you (or might not work at that point in the program). You may find that you can eat a particular food and have no reaction, whereas the person sitting next to you might notice a flare-up of symptoms if she or he eats it too often. This may have nothing to do with whether the food itself feeds candida, and more to do with your own unique physiology, medical history, or the current state of your intestinal microbiome. For better or worse, this same concept is true for every food you eat, even those in Stage 1. Each person is different, and not everyone can eat the same foods and still feel well. So, as with all things, pay attention—if you notice a particular reaction after eating a certain food, eliminate the suspects from your diet, at least temporarily.

reduction of candida in the system even more by including as many of the following specifically anticandida foods, in your menus as often as possible.

I try to eat at least a few of the foods from this list every day. Try to incorporate them more often than other foods (provided you're not allergic to them and they work for your body, of course).

Coconut oil: Coconut contains caprylic acid and monolaurin, both powerful antifungals. You can use the oil, which is the most powerful source of the antifungal properties, in smoothies, to make Homemade Chocolate (page 205), to sauté, roast vegetables, and so on. But any form of unsweetened coconut (coconut butter, shredded or fresh coconut) will deliver some of these substances and is good to eat, too.

Garlic: Garlic is another broad-spectrum antimicrobial that works well against candida. It's also a natural antibiotic, but, unlike prescription antibiotics, garlic doesn't kill the "good" bacteria, so it's safe to eat every day. Garlic's allicin compounds provide its anticandida properties, but these are killed by heat, so be sure to try to get some raw garlic if you can. I like to add one small clove to my fresh juices—you won't taste it in the juice, but it will boost the anticandida properties. If you can't tolerate it fresh, use a garlic supplement.

Pumpkin seeds: These green gems are antiparasitic and also help support the immune system with zinc, the mineral that's used in more bodily processes than any other. I include pumpkin seeds in many of the recipes in this book. Sprinkle raw or toasted seeds on salads, add them to smoothies, make homemade pumpkin seed milk (recipe on page 97), and so on.

Lemon and lime juice: Lemon and lime are not only great sources of vitamin C, they're also highly alkalizing. In addition, lemon supports the liver, which is likely working overtime while you're following the anticandida diet.

Naturally fermented foods: Naturally fermented (also called lacto-fermented) sauerkraut and kimchi, if made without sugars, can be incredibly useful as they repopulate the "friendly" gut bacteria (natural probiotics). In addition, naturally fermented foods such as these contain up to one hundred times more probiotics, as well as more different probiotic strains, than any probiotic capsules you buy. And the bonus? They're less expensive, and taste great! Start small (with about 1 to 2 teaspoons [5 to 10 ml]) per day, and build up to ¼ cup (60 ml) per day. Other naturally fermented foods include tempeh, miso, and natto.

Psyllium husks: The name may not be familiar, but you've likely heard of Metamucil, a product made from psyllium. Psyllium is a plant-based fiber that absorbs liquids and becomes gel-like when mixed with water. It supports detoxification by absorbing toxins in the body, then sweeping them out as it moves through the digestive tract and out of the body via elimination. It's also a great replacement for the gluten in gluten-free or grain-free baking, so you'll see it in many of my recipes, too (see page 81 for more on psyllium).

Chia seeds: These small, white or gray superfood seeds have been touted for their content of incredible omega-3 fatty acids (more than is found in flax), an essential nutrient that helps support a healthy immune system. They're also a great source of soluble fiber and contain amino acids that can help repair cell membranes. One of my favorite breakfasts or snacks is Basic Chia Pudding (page 101).

Highly alkaline foods: It's known that an acid-forming diet allows candida to thrive. By keeping the diet more alkaline, you encourage the yeast to take a hike and find another comfy home outside your body. Some of the best alkalizing foods are lemons; dark leafy greens, such as kale, collards, dandelion, spinach, and arugula; as well as other vegetables and fruits. Vegetable-based green juices made from wheatgrass, cucumber, and celery as major ingredients are also alkalizing. Of all grains, millet is the only one considered alkalizing, which may be why it's often included in anticandida diets (it's also usually nonallergenic).[1]

Chlorella: Not technically a "food," as it's rarely an ingredient on its own, chlorella is still an edible algae that can do wonders for your immune system and help with detoxification.[2] Add a bit to smoothies, salad dressings, or morning cereal.

A Note About Supplements

Antifungal supplements, digestive aids, prescription antifungals, and others are used by most practitioners in conjunction with a health-supportive diet that will help diminish the candida in your body. For each stage, work in consultation with your practitioner to determine which supplements and/or prescription antifungals you should take. For more on this, along with suggestions, please see pages 58–61.

Meals on the Diet: Set Plans or Make-Your-Own

If you're the kind of person who prefers to follow a preset menu plan, you'll find them on page 62. However, if you're more like me and like to use the plan as a guide but sometimes skip the listed meal for one you'd rather eat that night, feel free to use any recipes (or create your own) that fit within the dietary guidelines.

However, keep in mind that a candida-busting meal should generally contain all three of fat, fiber, and protein to keep your blood sugar balanced and prevent proliferation of yeast or cravings.

Optional "Fast Track"

The Fast Track version of the diet may be introduced any time after the first two weeks, and anytime within the later stages as a boost to your progress on the diet.

The Fast Track is a more challenging version of the diet, with additional food restrictions, and can be used whenever you wish to speed up the process; anytime you feel you've slipped (say, after a vacation) and need a "reboot"; or if your symptoms worsen at any point.

Even after six years on maintenance, for instance, I sometimes revert to the Fast Track after a period of traveling if I feel as if my diet hasn't been as clean as it should be. I will then remove grains for a week or two, which usually serves to quell any carb cravings that may have been reawakened during my time away from home. Then, once my eating habits return to normal, I allow grains back in.

Although it generates quicker results, the Fast Track is a more difficult diet to follow. To Fast Track at any point, simply remove one or more of the following ingredient groups from the basic diet (pages 41–44), for a period of one or more weeks (and up to three months at a time before reassessing):

- All grains, even gluten-free ones
- Sweet and starchy vegetables, such as beets, winter squashes, and all potatoes, even red-skinned ones

Please note: I don't believe it's necessary to pursue the Fast Track so as to heal from candida. Your progress may be more slow and steady if you retain some grains and the permitted starchy vegetables in your diet, but you will nevertheless heal over time. The dramatic, long-term changes will simply ensue more gradually, but they *will* happen if you stick with it.

In my case, I never moved to the Fast Track during the first year on the diet. My symptoms still resolved; and for me, continuing to use grains and as many vegetables as possible made sense given that I spend a lot of time in recipe development, food-based business, and social situations. So, while your progress may speed up on the Fast Track, choose your diet according to your own preferences and what makes sense for your lifestyle.

Stages of the Anticandida Diet

Many diets offer a separate stage to reintroduce some previously eaten foods and end there. My feeling is that, after an initial period of progress on the diet, broadening the acceptable food list should be a gradual process, and your body's reactions will let you know which foods you can tolerate and which you can't. For instance, in my case, I am able now (after six years on this plan) to tolerate the occasional (once a week, maximum twice a week) dessert that's made with "ACD-friendly" ingredients (such as those I used in my book *Naturally Sweet & Gluten-Free*). However, if I overdo it and continue to eat that way over several days, I may see a flare-up of symptoms again. If I revert to the "Fast Track" version of the diet once more at that point and consume a very clean, grain-free diet for a week or two, it disappears once again and I feel fine. You, too, will discover a balance that works for you.

Here are the different stages of the diet as I followed it, and what worked for me so I can maintain an overall sense of health without a recurrence of my symptoms.

Stage 1: The First 2 to 3 Months

What it is: Stage 1 is designed to remove as much of the excess yeast as possible, as quickly as possible, so your body can begin to heal. Always begin with at least two weeks of the basic diet as described on pages 41–44, then continue for up to three months before reassessing. Work in consultation with your practitioner to determine which supplements and/or prescription antifungals you should take during Stage 1.

How long it lasts: Initially, I'd recommend remaining on Stage 1 until you feel as if your worst symptoms have either disappeared or subsided significantly, usually a minimum of two to three months. Depending on the severity of your symptoms and how long you've been dealing with candida, you may not require that much time (or you may need longer; I was at this stage for four to six months).

What to look for before moving to Stage 2: You should notice major changes in symptoms or how you feel overall during this stage; ideally, your Yeast Assessment score will move to a lower category, or there will be major improvement. If you feel as if your condition has improved dramatically—or if what you considered your worst symptom has all but disappeared—then wait until your general condition remains stable (no further changes, and your score remains the same or improves) for at least three months before attempting to reintroduce some previously banned foods.

While I was following Stage 1, for example, the rash that had plagued me every moment diminished enough that, instead of itching 24 hours a day, I felt only a mild itchiness two or three times per day, and for a much shorter time (maybe a minute or so). The color faded from angry red to light pink, and the surface area shrank to about half what it had when I first began the diet. During this time, my constant cravings also subsided, so that I found myself seeking out sweet foods only occasionally each week instead of several times a day.

Stage 2: 4 or More Months on the Diet

What it is: After your symptoms have remained stable for a minimum of three months, Stage 2 continues with the diet but reintroduces some foods that have previously been banned. As with Stage 1, you should work in consultation with your practitioner to determine which supplements and/or prescription antifungals you should take, and which you can reduce or eliminate at this point. At this stage, your symptoms should be much less noticeable (or entirely gone), and your health dramatically improved as compared to when you began the diet. Look for your Yeast Assessment score to shift lower, ideally moving to "Mild & Manageable" or "Moderate & Malleable."

Once you feel your condition is stable (no further changes, and your score remains the same or improves) for at least three months, begin by bringing back one food at a time, eating it once and then waiting a couple of days to see whether you have a flare-up of your symptom(s). If there are no changes after a week, try introducing another food at this point, until all the allowed Stage 2 foods that you desire have been reintroduced.

What to reintroduce: It's best to reintroduce no more than one new food at a time, then wait two to four days to see whether your body has a reaction. If so, remove that food again; if not and things continue to be well, choose a new food the following week, and so on.

Begin to reintroduce whole foods, such as:

- "Nonsweet" fruits, such as apples, pears, peaches; plus fresh pineapple and fresh papaya (though sweet, they contain natural digestive enzymes and so are acceptable here): no more than one per day
- Some grain-based or pseudo-grain flours and gluten-free grains (I reintroduced sorghum, teff, and amaranth as well as some gluten-free flours); at Stage 2, some people can also tolerate certified gluten-free oats
- Unsweetened, organic 100 percent cacao chocolate (in addition to raw cacao powder)

How long it lasts: Once your symptoms have improved to the point that you feel (mostly) well again, it's a good idea to continue at the same stage for a minimum of three more months to ensure that your health is stable. I would always wait about three months before I attempted to reintroduce Stage 3 foods at any point.

What to look for before moving to Stage 3: During Stage 2, your body is adjusting to a new way of eating and is still repairing long-term damage. While you will feel much, much better than you did at the beginning and may even think your candida is completely gone, there may be more healing required before you can reintroduce foods that you used to eat before you began the ACD.

During this stage, I felt confident that my candida was entirely under control and was raring to begin using my old favorite ingredients again. My rash was no longer visible, my foggy thinking was gone, and I felt more energetic than I had in years. As I began to introduce certain foods, however, I noticed that too much of any one ingredient (say, a baked good for breakfast one day, pasta the next, a homemade bread a couple of days later) could still trigger symptoms. I scaled back, took care of my digestion and my immune system, and eventually was stable again. For me, flour-based products are usually fine for up to two times a week; it may be different for you.

Note, too, that there is no need to reintroduce new foods at all if you're feeling great or you feel there is still more investigation needed to get you to your 100 percent recovery. Many people live for a lifetime within the parameters I've outlined here, feeling healthy and satisfied by their food.

Stage 3: 1 Year and Beyond

What it is: This is the maintenance stage of your ACD, how you'll likely eat for the rest of your days. The specific foods and beverages that you may consume at this stage will be different from mine or someone else's; this is the diet you'll follow to maintain good health and keep your candida from returning. As with the previous stages, you should work in consultation with your practitioner to determine which supplements and/or prescription antifungals you should take, and which you can reduce or eliminate at this point. To move to this stage, your Yeast Assessment score should be "Mild & Manageable" (ideally, with a score at the low end of this category).

What to reintroduce:
- A broader range of fruits (only occasionally). In Stage 3, it's okay to experiment with sweeter fruits, such as mango or pomegranate, or dried fruits with the lowest sugar content, such as goji berries, golden berries, or dried prunes. Dried fruits with the highest sugar content, such as raisins or dates, are normally avoided indefinitely (though, go ahead and experiment with them if you've been stable for a year or so—they may be okay for you).
- Prepared nut butters (100 percent nuts); I'll use ready-made nut butters only if they contain nothing but organic nuts (or, occasionally, organic oils); however, remember to avoid peanut butter.
- "Dead" yeasts (e.g., in bread or nutritional yeast); avoid these if you have an allergic reaction);
- Some regular salad vinegars (e.g., balsamic or rice vinegar); I generally still avoid these in maintenance but will have them if they're part of a restaurant salad, for instance.
- Infrequently, treats made with low-glycemic natural sweeteners (e.g., coconut sugar, coconut nectar, agave syrup, or brown rice syrup). I will occasionally enjoy a treat (e.g., a cookie or other homemade baked good) made with one of these sweeteners, usually cutting the sweetener with stevia to lower the overall glycemic index of the confection. These should be consumed judiciously and seen as rare exceptions for special occasions; definitely no more than once per week.

How long it lasts: This is the diet you should plan to follow indefinitely. I followed this stage for at least six months before considering whether to add even more foods to my diet plan.

What to look for before moving on: Generally, you can look at minor additions to this stage after a minimum of six months of stability eating this way. At that point, I'd consider adding further to the range of food and drink, but only rarely or on very special occasions.

So, for instance, you might wish to have a few sips of wine at your birthday, or consume a dessert with dates at a special occasion; but beware—adding back foods with such high sugar content is a slippery slope, and it's all too easy to begin consuming (and craving) them on a regular basis again—potentially triggering the candida overgrowth all over. Again, I'd introduce only one food at a time, then wait three or four days to ensure that you don't have an adverse reaction before welcoming that food back into your diet.

After the Diet: Long-Term Maintenance

As you continue to thrive on your anticandida lifestyle, you may wish to consume foods from your previous diet or new foods that come out on the market.

As a general rule when deciding which foods I can or cannot try, I look at the quality of the food (is it a whole food? organic? non-GMO? etc.) as well as the glycemic index and/or glycemic load of the food. If something is low on the glycemic index, it's not likely to spike my blood sugar levels, so I am more willing to give it a try than if it contains sugar or other refined ingredients.

Foods That Should Never Be Part of a Healthy Diet

That said, there are certain foods I would never (*ever, ever!*) reintroduce to my diet, not only because they can trigger candida overgrowth in a heartbeat, but because they are, frankly, unhealthy in any case.

This is the list of foods you should really avoid for the rest of your life. Since 2009 I've not touched any food that contains these ingredients, and I see no reason to ever eat them again.

- White (refined) sugar or any type of cane sugar, including organic sugar, raw sugar, evaporated cane juice, etc.
- Refined white all-purpose wheat flour or any non-gluten-free flour
- Hydrogenated oils (margarine, "buttery spread," etc.)
- Moldy foods (e.g., blue cheeses) and mushrooms, except the occasional medicinal mushrooms (reishi, chaga, etc.)

- Excessive alcohol. The definition of *excessive* will vary depending on your metabolism and tolerance. In general, I wouldn't imbibe more than one glass of wine or liquor every couple of weeks or so (though, in reality, I don't even drink that much); this amount may differ for you. Your body is the best guide to what can or can't be tolerated.

As you can see, even with these "restricted" food lists, you will still be eating a broad, whole foods–based diet from which you can prepare delicious, enticing recipes. Most important, remember that this diet will help free you from the grip that candida has over your body and your health. With that thought in mind, you can relish every bite, knowing that you are doing something truly beneficial for yourself!

Other Food Considerations

Because so many variations of the anticandida diet are out there, you may have encountered versions that permit certain foods not on this list or veto other foods that are. Why are some foods allowed in some cases, while others are not? That question alone was a major reason I took a sabbatical from the college where I taught to study holistic nutrition at the Canadian School of Natural Nutrition! I remember wondering, "If it's a natural, whole food that doesn't contain sugar, what could be wrong—right?" Well, not always right.

Following is my own perspective on some of the more controversial foods in my "yes" list, or those that are sometimes deemed acceptable and sometimes not in other diets. As always, you should make your own choices based on your individual situation, in consultation with your own doctor or health-care provider.

Soy Products

The debate over soy has been raging for some time in nutrition circles and seems it's still not entirely resolved: is soy a healthy, nourishing superfood, or is it a hormone-disrupting, digestion-damaging "Frankenfood" to be avoided at all costs? As with all topics sensationalized in the media, the answer likely lies somewhere in between.

Ever since the FDA recommended consuming 25 grams of soy products daily as a way to reduce risk of heart disease, it seems as if the mass marketing of soy products—*any* soy products—has burgeoned. Yet in recent years, studies have suggested that soy products can interfere with proper digestion (because they contain protease inhibitors, phytates, oxalates, and other substances that make them difficult to digest); that they may contribute to breast cancer; that they interfere with proper thyroid functioning (because they contain goitrogens); or that they contain phytoestrogens (plant estrogens) that interfere with or block natural estrogen.[3] In addition, most of the commercially produced soy in North America is genetically modified, and we don't yet have long-term data as to whether this fiddling with nature will prove harmful to humans' health. On the other hand, many experts still recommend soy as a healthful food, citing opposing studies that demonstrate how it helps prevent breast cancer or other cancers.[4]

As you can see from the "Foods to Eat Freely" list, I recommend soy on the anticandida diet. To date, I have not found any major studies arguing against the use of fermented soy products (e.g., tempeh, miso, or tamari) because the fermenting process reduces the antidigestion toxins, such as phytates and oxalates; and, because soy really is one of the best sources of plant-based protein, containing sufficient amounts of all essential amino acids, I think fermented soy should be included in a healthy vegan diet. Please be sure that your soy is either organic (by default, non-GMO) or clearly labeled as "non-GMO," however!

Raw Cacao and Cocoa

When I first started the anticandida diet back in 1999, I remember being overwrought with despair, thinking, "No more milk chocolate? Not *ever*? Will life still be worth living? . . ." Of course, the correct answers to those questions are, respectively, "No more," "No, not ever," and "Of course, silly!"

But don't despair! That doesn't mean you can never enjoy chocolate at all. If you're a chocolate devotee like I am, you probably already know that chocolate is considered a superfood, brimming with antioxidants that can help prevent heart disease.[5] The key to remember here, however, is that those studies refer to pure, dark chocolate. Most bars you purchase in the grocery store—or even the health food store—are highly processed and made with alkalized (Dutch-processed) cocoa; but the alkalizing process itself removes most of the beneficial antioxidants. They also contain sugar in one form or another.

In other words, if you wish to enjoy chocolate on the ACD, it's best to use raw cacao powder (ground raw cacao beans, from which chocolate is made), mix it into a form of homemade chocolate with cacao butter or coconut oil, and sweeten to taste yourself with stevia (see recipe, page 205). Another reason why I prefer raw cacao is that I find the flavor much less bitter than that of commercial cocoa powder, and it's easier to reach a palatable level of sweetness by using stevia as the only sweetener.

But take note: Even raw cacao can trigger cravings, so it may not be your best choice in the early stages of the diet. It also contains caffeine, which some suggest can trigger cravings as well.[6] I recommend waiting until you feel stable for at least a month, then trying one dessert recipe with cacao and monitoring your reaction. If you find yourself craving it or consuming an entire batch of brownies in a day, you may still be too close to the allure of cacao to use it just yet.

In my case, I cut out all cacao or chocolate for the first few months of the diet, until my cravings had subsided and I felt better able to handle it; until then, I used carob as a substitute. No, it doesn't taste exactly like chocolate, but it has a lovely, sweet flavor all its own.

Grains or No Grains? Legumes or No Legumes?

Some anticandida diets prohibit all grains or legumes throughout the program or most of the program. For instance, *The Body Ecology Diet* suggests initially cutting out all legumes (because they are "too difficult to digest, and they cause fermentation and sugars")[7] as well as most grains because they feed the yeast.[8] Grains are often prohibited because of their high carbohydrate content (which ultimately converts to sugar via digestion). For instance, Drs. Levin and Gare's diet[9] eliminates almost all carbohydrates in the early stages of the diet. Others, such as Whole Approach,[10] allow some grains and legumes right from the beginning.

The diet I present here offers you many gluten-free grains as well as all legumes except peas, which contain high amounts of sugar. Beans and legumes are wonderful sources of protein on a vegan diet; they also contain a natural combination of protein and starch in a single food designed by nature to house both those nutrients. Whole grains contain many important nutrients, a good amount of fiber, and some protein as well. I feel that they are a healthful choice, and, with a low glycemic index (GI), neither of these foods should spike blood sugar levels when you consume them as part of your overall meal. For that reason, you'll find them in these menus and recipes.

What you won't find in the early stages, however, are grain-based, or even pseudo-grain (e.g., quinoa or teff) flours. Flour is a processed food. Even if it's made from whole grains without anything added or subtracted, grinding up whole grains exposes the interior (where the natural oils are housed) to air and light, encouraging oxidation and reduction of the nutrient qualities. I prefer whole grains for the same reason I prefer whole nuts or seeds with the shells still on—they remain fresher, longer.

Nuts—Which Are Acceptable?

Most anticandida diets strongly prohibit peanuts and pistachios because of their high mold contents. (In fact, I haven't been able to find a single version of the diet that does allow either one of these.) Most commonly, conventional peanuts (as well as other crops, particularly corn) can be afflicted with toxins called aflatoxins, which are a specific by-product of certain molds that can do serious damage to the liver and kidneys over time.[11] Apparently, it's impossible to eradicate all traces of these mycotoxins in foods, so their numbers are strictly monitored by most government agencies to ensure that they don't pose a safety risk to most people.

According to the organization Food Safety Watch, foods known to be at the highest risk for aflatoxins are "maize [corn], groundnuts (peanuts), pistachios, brazils, chillies, black pepper, dried fruit and figs."[12]

Given the fact that most other nuts may or may not contain aflatoxins but are nevertheless excluded from the "highest-mold" category, it made sense to me to follow my naturopath's advice and consume other nuts in moderation, particularly on a vegan diet where nuts are an important source of protein and healthy fats. As always, please see what works best for you and stick with that.

Do note, however, that most commercially roasted nuts are coated in cheap, most likely rancid oils and should never be consumed. If you wish to eat nuts as a snack, buy whole, raw nuts (preferably organic) in bulk and then toast them at 350°F (180°C) for about 10 minutes, until fragrant (or, better yet, soak and dehydrate them first if you're able; see the instructions on pages 95 and 97).

"Shortcut" Foods

When you're just starting out, and as a time-saving device, it makes sense to rely on shortcuts if they help keep you on program.

Nondairy milks: While I'd prefer that all milks be homemade, go ahead and use the packaged ones if they fit within the dietary guidelines (unsweetened, all natural) and will prevent you from veering off course. I find that the best alternative milks are almond and hemp.

Nut and seed butters: Once you've made your own nut butter and see how easy it is to create (and how superior the taste), you may never go back. However, if you don't have time to process your own, buying all-natural nut and seed butters (they should contain one ingredient—whatever the nut or seed is) is a fine alternative. Remember that natural nut and seed butters must be refrigerated once they are opened; unlike most commercial peanut butters, they don't contain sugar or preservatives to prevent degradation at room temperature.

Protein powder: While legumes, nuts, seeds, greens, and grains all provide decent amounts of protein, you may sometimes find you need a boost or wish to add more protein to prevent blood sugar spikes. A good protein powder should contain as few ingredients as possible with no additives or chemicals. Growing Naturals pea protein boasts one single ingredient (yellow pea protein);[13] similarly, Vega hemp protein contains only that, hemp protein.

Canned foods: If you can find canned goods that contain just simple ingredients (and only one or two of them) in BPA-free cans, these are, in a pinch, acceptable choices on the ACD. You'll see that a few of the recipes (e.g., the Quick and Easy Chard and Chickpea Soup, page 149, or Eggplant "Parmesan," page 192) call for canned tomatoes for this very reason. Try to keep canned goods to a minimum, no more than twice a week, however.

Supplements: Antifungals and More

As I noted earlier, antifungal supplements, digestive aids, prescription antifungals, and others are used by most practitioners in conjunction with a health-supportive diet that will help diminish the candida in your body. As you undoubtedly know by now, however, each person comprises a unique set of genetics and circumstances, so what worked for me may or may not work exactly the same way for you.

Following is a list of the most useful supplements and antifungals that I used or have encountered over the years.

The protocol I followed included some of these supplements at each stage of the diet. However, before you incorporate any of these into your own anticandida diet, please check with your health-care practitioner to ensure that they are also right for you. Even though these substances (except for prescription drugs) are "natural" and available over the counter, keep in mind that even natural supplements can contain powerful chemicals and compounds that act like drugs in the system; in other words, always be mindful of possible interactions or overuse, so use them correctly, and please don't try any of these without professional supervision. Your health-care provider will be able to help you with correct dosages.

Antifungals

Antifungals are used to kill the yeast and related organisms.

Oral

- Oil of oregano
- Caprylic acid, lauric acid, monolaurin (these substances are all derived from coconut oil, so you can acquire a certain amount by eating coconut and coconut oil; for more concentrated amounts, supplements can be used)
- Cloves or clove tea
- Grapefruit seed (citrus seed) extract
- Black walnut
- Garlic (fresh is best, but you can use supplements as well)
- Pomegranate husk
- Goldenseal (should never be used long term)
- Olive leaf extract
- Grapeseed extract
- Pau d'arco (decoction)
- Wormwood
- Colloidal silver (can become toxic over time—*always* use under professional supervision!)
- systemic enzymes (nattokinase, serrapeptase)
- RX: nystatin, Diflucan, clotrimazole

Topical
- Boric acid[14] (must be diluted to use on skin)
- Gentian violet
- Tea tree oil (*must* be diluted to use on skin)
- Oil of oregano (*must* be diluted to use on skin)
- Grapefruit seed extract (*must* be diluted to use on skin)
- RX: nystatin, clotrimazole, myconazole

Improve digestion and Heal Leaky Gut

- L-glutamine
- Cabbage juice[15]
- Aloe vera juice
- Magnesium
- Slippery elm
- Digestive enzymes (look for brands that have amylase, protease, and lipase at a minimum)
- *Saccharomyces boulardii*

Boost and Support the Immune System

- Probiotics (fermented foods are a great source, or use a supplement with at least several billion active cells)
- Vitamin B complex
- Raw apple cider vinegar
- Zinc
- Flaxseeds (also good for removing toxins and for essential fatty acids)
- Milk thistle
- Nettle tea
- Multivitamins
- Dandelion tea
- Astragalus
- Echinacea

Remove Toxins from the Body

- Bentonite clay or diatomaceous earth (*must* be food grade)
- Psyllium husk
- Ground flax or chia seeds
- Cilantro[16]
- Blue-green algae (e.g., chlorella or spirulina)[17]

A note about probiotics: Although some practitioners suggest that reintroducing probiotics in Stage 1 is too early (because many of the supplements designed to kill candida will also kill off the probiotics), I believe that some of the probiotic strains will still survive and can help repopulate gut bacteria even as the yeast dies off. Consequently, I suggest taking probiotics throughout the entire diet (just be sure to take them at least two hours away from other supplements).

Sample Meal Plans

Following are separate meal plans for Stage 1 and Stage 2. I haven't included a sample plan for Stage 3, since that is maintenance; at that point, you will be adding back foods as your health and wellness allows. Do note, however, that you're welcome to eat any of the listed recipes at any meal, add your own recipes, or repeat certain recipes more than once if you prefer those and not others. The only real "rule" is to stay within the food list according to the level and stage of the diet you're currently following.

Note that these recipes do include grains and legumes. If you follow the "Fast Track" version of the diet, you may need to repeat more recipes that are nut-based to avoid those ingredients.

Other notes:

- You can always add extra salad or vegetables to any of the meals (including breakfast!).
- I try to consume lacto-fermented sauerkraut at least once a day with a meal.
- I've included either one snack or dessert per day, as I avoid eating dessert every day. If you're feeling like you need one, go ahead and have one of the ACD-friendly desserts more often.

Stage 1 Sample Menu

	BREAKFAST	LUNCH	DINNER	SNACKS
MONDAY	ACD-Friendly Grain-Free Granola (page 123) with dairy-free milk of choice	Roasted Garlic and Cauliflower Soup (page 147) with Grain-Free Sandwich Bread (page 102) or leftover (from Sunday) ACD Whole-Grain Waffle (page 119) and Creamy Kale Salad with Black Beans and Sweet Potato (page 170)	Zucchini Linguine with Lentil-Tomato Sauce (page 200) and Caesar Salad (page 175)	Raw Carrot Cake Energy Balls (page 142)
TUESDAY	Sweet Potato Rounds with Sweet or Savory Almond Sauce (page 129)	Creamy Broccoli Soup (page 150) with leftover Caesar Salad (page 175) and Grain-Free Sandwich Bread (page 102)	Pumpkin Patties (page 187); Cauliflower and Bean Mash (page 137) and green salad	"Sour Cream and Onion" Kale Chips (page 139)
WEDNESDAY	"It Is the ONE" Single-Serve Pancake (page 121) with nut butter topping	Vegetable Miso Soup (page 146) with Raw Sushi with Spicy Ginger-Miso Sauce (page 183)	Chickpea "Quiche" (page 186) with green salad	Crimson Mousse (page 215)
THURSDAY	Smooth Operator Smoothie (page 114)	Curried Carrot-Lentil Soup (page 145) with Crimson Salad (page 164) and Grain-Free Sandwich Bread (page 102)	Veggie Fried Quinoa with Arame and Edamame (page 195)	Sweet and Spicy Roasted Chickpeas (page 138)
FRIDAY	Chia-Rice Pudding (page 128) or Basic Chia Pudding (page 101) with nut butter swirled into it if desired; Mojito Smoothie (page 115)	Asian Napa Cabbage Salad (page 168) with My Favorite Hummus (page 161) and Zucchini Chips (page 141)	Grain-Free Pizza (page 104) with Broccoli-Lemon Pesto (page 181), Oven-Dried Tomatoes (page 106), and Meaty Crumbles (page 107); plus Cabbage and Broccoli Slaw (page 163)	S'Mores Parfaits (page 217)
SATURDAY	Veggie-Full Breakfast Hash (page 131) grilled tomatoes; and Almond-Crusted Root Vegetable "Fries" (page 135)	Leftover pizza	Super Stuffed Sweet Potatoes (page 185) with As-You-Like Kale Salad (page 172)	Grain-Free Fudgy Brownies (page 206)
SUNDAY	(Brunch) Fluffy Pancakes (page 120) or ACD Whole-Grain Waffles (page 119) with nut butter of choice and Coconut-Cranberry Spread (page 158), plus Rutabaga "Hash Browns" (page 132)		Sunday Night Roast (page 196) with Perfect Golden Gravy (page 177); broccoli or other green vegetable; and Almond-Crusted Root Vegetable "Fries" (page 135)	Vanilla Ice Cream (page 220)

Stage 2 Sample Menu

Note the addition of fruits.

	BREAKFAST	LUNCH	DINNER	SNACKS/DESSERT
MONDAY	Raw Apple Porridge Bowl (page 125) with Grain-Free Sandwich Bread (page 102) or leftover Whole Grain Waffles (page 119) [from Sunday previous]	Grain and Veggie Meal-in-a-Bowl (page 201)	Herbed Grain-Free Gnocchi (page 188) in Fresh Spicy Tomato Sauce, (page 180) with As-You-Like Kale Salad (page 172)	Avocado Mousse (page 214)
TUESDAY	Classic Green Smoothie (page 113)	Chunky Black Bean Spread (page 159) with raw veggies and Grain-Free Sandwich Bread (page 102)	Veggie Fried Quinoa with Arame and Edamame (page 195); Asian Napa Cabbage Salad (page 168)	"Sour Cream and Onion" Kale Chips (page 139)
WEDNESDAY	Zucchini Fritters (page 129) with Garlicky Warm Avocado Sauce (page 179) or Savory Almond Sauce (page 178)	Creamy Broccoli Soup (page 150) with leftover Asian Napa Cabbage Salad (page 168)	Grain-Free Pizza (page 104) with Broccoli-Lemon Pesto (page 181), Oven-Dried Tomatoes (page 106), and Meaty Crumbles (page 107), plus Caesar Salad (page 175)	Raw veggies with leftover Chunky Black Bean Spread (page 159)
THURSDAY	ACD-Friendly Grain-Free Granola (page 123) with homemade nut or seed milk (page 97)	Curried Carrot-Lentil Soup (page 145) with leftover Caesar Salad (page 175, or any green salad)	Creamy Black Beans and Rutabaga Stew (page 202) with Cabbage and Broccoli Slaw (page 163)	Zucchini Chips (page 141)
FRIDAY	Baked Quinoa Porridge (page 126)	Creamy Kale Salad with Black Beans and Sweet Potato (page 170) with Grain-Free Sandwich Bread (page 102)	Tempeh "Bourguignon" (page 198) over brown rice or quinoa; broccoli or other veggie side, or salad of choice	Grain-Free Apple Berry Crumble (page 212)
SATURDAY	The "Toronto" Sandwich (page 151) with salad of choice	Beans Paprikash (page 191) over cooked buckwheat	Eggplant "Parmesan" (page 192) with Dandelion-Apple Salad (page 165)	Raw Frosted "Put the Lime in the Coconut" Bars (page 211)
SUNDAY	(Brunch): ACD Whole-Grain Waffles (page 119) with Glazed Tempeh (page 111) and Rutabaga "Hash Browns," (page 132) plus green salad of choice		Sunday Night Roast (page 196) with Perfect Golden Gravy (page 177); Cauliflower and Bean Mash (page 137); and Baby Greens with Pear and Walnuts in a Cranberry-Poppyseed Dressing (page 167)	Vanilla Ice Cream (page 220)

Fast Track Sample Menus

If you opt for the Fast Track and eliminate all grains and legumes, note that you will need to supplement with additional protein in most meals to replace them, for example, additional nuts or seeds.

	BREAKFAST	LUNCH	DINNER	SNACKS
DAY 1	Protein-Boost Cranberry Smoothie (page 116)	Raw Almond-Veggie Pâté with vegetables (page 160)	As-You-Like Kale Salad (page 172; omit fruit and sweet vegetables)	Zucchini Chips (page 141) or Avocado Mousse (page 214)
DAY 2	Almost Instant Grain-Free Breakfast Porridge (just omit fruit) (page 127)	Raw Sushi with Spicy Ginger-Miso Sauce (page 183); use allowed vegetables	Asian Napa Cabbage Salad (page 168; omit carrot)	"Sour Cream and Onion" Kale Chips (page 139) or Raw Frosted "Put the Lime in the Coconut" Bars (page 211)
DAY 3	Rutabaga "Hash Browns" (page 132)	Cabbage and Broccoli Slaw (page 163)	As-You-Like Kale Salad (page 172; omit fruit and sweet vegetables)	S'Mores Parfaits (page 217)

CHAPTER 4

Strategies for a Successful Anticandida Diet

So, how can you ensure that you're prepared—in practical terms as well as psychologically—to embark on this diet? Beginning an anticandida regime can be daunting, as it may mean a radical change in what you eat, dealing with ongoing cravings, navigating social and family situations, and more. But there's good news: armed with the right tools and techniques, you'll be ready to ace this hurdle! And again, if you're worried that the ACD is all about restriction and denial, rest assured that the recipes offered here are bountiful, delicious, and satisfying. There's no reason to feel deprived. Following are some of the most common challenges you may face, and what you can do about them.

Challenge 1: Preconceived Notions About the Diet (or, if you think you can or you think you can't—you're probably right)

I sometimes hear naturopathic doctors discuss matters of "patient compliance" related to an anticandida diet. One of my former practitioners even told me that the ACD was the most difficult diet for patients to follow, even harder than an allergy elimination diet.

If you're reading this book, you may have attempted one or more anticandida diets already. For many people, the biggest challenge is simply *getting started*; then, once you've begun, the second biggest challenge is staying on the diet *long enough* to see results.

And, as I did, many people who contemplate starting an anticandida diet put it off, often for the same reasons: "It's too strict. I'll never be able to follow it." "How will I live without all of my favorite foods?" "What will I do at social occasions? Will I have to avoid my friends for months until I get this candida under control?" or "Will I need to spend all of my time in the kitchen now that I'm on this diet?" I'm happy to report that all of those concerns can be addressed easily, starting with a subtle shift in attitude.

Yes, it's true that you won't be eating all the same foods that normally ate when you're following the anticandida diet. But that doesn't mean you won't enjoy your food just as much as you did before! I like to take the perspective of visiting a foreign country. I've never been to Greece, and I am quite sure that the food they eat on the other side of the Atlantic is markedly different from what I can find in my own home town. That said, I also have no doubt I'd love me some spanakopita, baklava, tzatziki, or any of the other native specialties (I'd seek out plant-based versions, of course).

The point is that *different* need not equal *unappealing*.

While on holidays, many of us are willing to sample foods we might not enjoy at any other time. Think of your anticandida diet as a holiday from the acidic, disease-promoting fast foods and processed foods that may have brought you to this point in the first place. And, just as you enjoyed the foods you've been accustomed to eating, you will come to love your ACD menu just as much.

After years of eating this way, I literally can't go more than a day without leafy greens, or my body begins to crave them. I love chia pudding with a passion, and I have grown to adore pure, dark chocolate just as much as I used to relish my cans of "milk chocolate" frosting—more, actually, since I know that the homemade version I eat nourishes and supports my good health, whereas the junk food products led me down the path to illness in the first place.

Remember that foods on the anticandida diet are all health-promoting, whole foods that will help your body fight the foreign invader that's making you sick. Isn't that fact alone enough reason to embrace it wholeheartedly?

Challenge 2: A Long List of New Foods

I clearly recall when I walked out of my ND's office after the first appointment about candida. My head was spinning: *What the heck is kale? What's quinoa? Who ever heard of tamari?* I had no idea. I scrambled to the health food store and relied on the sympathetic staff member to find everything for me. I was sure I'd dislike the flavors of these weird new "foods." And worst of all, I had to learn to *cook* with them!

No doubt, change is scary. We humans are creatures of habit and we tend to resist change. In fact, studies show that change causes stress, even when the change is a good one that the person may have sought out willingly.[1] When we're faced with a major transformation in our diet that we didn't particularly want or request, the transition can seem even more daunting.

But ironically, once you commit to change and adapt, that situation becomes the "new normal" and you can't imagine anything else. When you first get married and sport a wedding band, you may be acutely aware of it on your finger for a few days. It clicks when you open a door, it slides around over your knuckle, it glistens in the sun and distracts you as you drive home from work. Within a short time, however, your body adapts and you no longer realize it's even there. You've grown accustomed to the change and it's now your new normal.

I promise, this kind of adjustment will occur with this diet, too. I'm totally at home eating this way now and can't imagine anything else.

The same is true of these new foods. The foods on this diet truly nourish your body, so welcome them. And, as I mentioned before, the recipes in *Living Candida-Free* won't feel restrictive and will both look and taste familiar. As you'll see in the recipe section, you can still enjoy waffles, pancakes, bread, brownies, ice cream, fudge—even chocolate; they just won't contain identical ingredients to versions of those foods you ate before. (And trust me, once you've become accustomed to crisp, fresh kale; rich and silky homemade chocolate bars; hearty, robust whole-grain breakfast cereal or healthy, crunchy roasted chickpea snacks, your body will thank you and you'll discover that the old stuff really doesn't appeal anymore.)

It's also important to remember that some change is actually good. My parents grew up without computers; my father grew up on a farm without running water. Without change, we'd all still be living in caves and munching on berries or gnawing on freshly speared raw buffalo for dinner.

Challenge 3: Cravings

As you saw in Chapter 1, candida is a ravenous, demanding organism. As the yeast begins to die off, it will cry out for more food, and you may experience sometimes powerful urges to consume sugar or other foods.

Cravings are an inevitable part of the diet, and the more you prepare for them in advance, the more you can deal with them successfully.

As with biochemical reactions to medications, each body is unique, so cravings will affect each of us differently. Some people will demonstrate the classic pattern of cravings that appear and dissipate within a week of starting a sugar-free diet; others (such as myself) will take longer to reboot their metabolism so that cravings become a thing of the past. Whatever your situation, there are ways to ensure that the cravings don't sabotage your success at conquering candida.

To begin with, identifying the different kinds of cravings can be a useful tool in your arsenal of tactics to neutralize them. For instance, many cravings appear because of irregularities in blood sugar or nutrient deficiencies, and we can easily remedy that situation through carefully planning when and what to eat (such as always including fat, fiber, and protein in every meal or snack). Other cravings are associated with emotional or psychological factors and may require longer-term approaches or a different perspective that allows us to accept the cravings and move on.

Either way, here are some of the most effective approaches I've found over the years to quash cravings, especially when you first begin the diet and the call of sugar can feel overwhelming.

1. Tap Into Your Inner Girl (or Boy) Scout

One of the most reliable tactics for avoiding cravings is to be prepared for them. Stock your home with ACD-friendly foods and remove anything that could sabotage your diet. That way, you won't be tempted to eat something that might encourage yeast to stick around (or, at the least, you'll make it that much more difficult to acquire those foods). If you live with other people who are not on the diet, you can ask them to hide the "taboo" foods that might tempt you.

2. Remember That "No" Is Easier Than "Maybe"

In her online sugar detox and blood sugar balancing program that I help Andrea teach, she refers to this concept as "staying on the path." As she notes, for each of us there are certain behaviors that are simply never considered within the realm of what we'd actually do; they are nonnegotiable. So, for instance, most of us never smoke crack cocaine; it's beyond the average person's reality. Most of us don't rob banks, beat up little children, or tattoo our nose. Similarly, you can decide that consuming sugar is one of those nonnegotiable activities.

Over the years, I've been tempted by many foods; and as I've continued to heal, I've allowed many previously verboten ingredients, such as balsamic vinegar or dates, back into my diet on occasion. But white sugar has never been a consideration. It's simply a "no" food. And knowing that I don't ever have to think about it makes my decision to avoid it that much easier.

3. Practice "Safe Binges"

When I'm feeling the need for something sweet, I often mix up a small batch of something—say, a recipe of Emergency Fudge (page 208). In that case, I know that even if I let loose and consume the entire batch, I haven't done my ACD, or my health, any harm. These treats contain healthful ingredients and won't wreak havoc with my blood sugar levels to ultimately sabotage my success (which could lead to further cravings). The worst that will happen is that my caloric intake for the day will be slightly higher than usual.

Making a small batch also prevents me from eating beyond those few pieces because it would feel like too much trouble to subsequently mix up a new recipe after the first one is finished (I'm inherently lazy like that). So, go ahead and mix up small portions of your trigger foods, then stop when they're gone. It's a good idea to have some "safe" treats in the freezer for just this type of situation.

4. It's Easier Being Green

Yeast thrives in an acidic environment, and green foods promote alkalinity in the body. Eating "green" has been one of my most important tactics to suppress or eliminate sweet cravings. When I consume a lot of leafy greens and other alkalizing foods, my cravings simply never make an appearance.

Along those lines, I've noticed if I start my day with a savory breakfast, I tend not to crave sweet things later on in the day. Donna Gates in *Body Ecology* recommends a bit of water with raw apple cider vinegar (with stevia as a sweetener) as a cravings buster; that drink is also very alkalizing. The ACD-Friendly Fruity Sipper (page 116) is a variation on this idea, and is something I enjoy several times each week.

5. Strategic Procrastination

Years ago, I edited a book of essays, one of which described a woman's experiences learning to become a successful student. Her method was to promise herself she'd sit down and practice the piano for just ten minutes, even when she didn't feel like it; and she set a timer for that amount of time. She knew that only ten minutes was doable and wouldn't feel onerous. Inevitably, once the timer went off, she had already become involved in her playing and wanted to keep going.

Similarly, it's a good idea to set a mental (or real) timer for twenty minutes anytime you feel a strong food craving; then concentrate on a different task in the interim. Once the timer goes off, check in again with your craving. You may find that it has already dissipated, or you may have discovered what it is you're truly craving instead. (And if the craving is still there? See "Practice Safe Binges," page 69).

6. Balance the Blood Sugar Tightrope with Ease

One of the very best methods to prevent cravings entirely is to ensure that blood sugar levels remain stable and that you don't spike insulin production by eating foods with a high-glycemic load. This means including the key trio of fat, fiber, and protein at each meal or snack to not only provide all the macronutrients you need but also ensure that the overall glycemic load of your food won't cause blood sugar peaks and valleys that can initiate cravings.

In other words, if you consume a sweet treat, be sure to pair it with protein, fiber, or fat (or all three, depending on what's already in the treat). To take the guess work out for you, the snack and dessert recipes in this book already provide a good mix of these three nutrients.

And while we're talking about nutrients: Note that all carbohydrates are not the same! The term *carbohydrate* refers to pretty much any plant food, and technically "carbs" are one or more of sugars, starches, or fiber. For our purposes, I focus on fiber (e.g., as found in whole grains, legumes, and vegetables), or carbohydrates that appear as natural starches (e.g., those in grains or legumes). I try to limit the sugars in the foods we eat as much as possible, since those feed the candida.

Because starches are quickly converted to sugars in the body, pure starches (e.g., cornstarch, tapioca starch, arrowroot, potato starch) are used sparingly, if at all, to limit their effect on blood glucose levels. On the other hand, fiber can't be digested by the human body, so it acts as a bulk-builder that not only keeps us regular but also (in the form of inulin, sometimes called prebiotics) feeds the good bacteria that we want to rebuild in the gut. In other words, eat a lot of fiber! Fiber is great to flush out toxins as well, something you'll want to do while on the diet.

7. Acknowledge and Move On

One of the greatest food revelations for me was that I could acknowledge cravings without having to act on them. I now think of cravings as a physical reaction that manifests without my conscious permission. Just like any other minor (and unwanted) interruption in my day, such as a ringing telephone or rain against the windowpane, I can consciously note the craving without responding to it.

Several years ago, I participated in a cleanse led by one of my instructors from nutrition school. During one session, she addressed the issue of emotional baggage we all carry around. At the end of the class, she remarked, "You may still feel hungry after you eat some of these meals. Now, understand that your nutritional needs are being met, and your body doesn't actually need more food. So, if you feel hungry, it's a different kind of hunger you're feeling—emotional, or psychological. Know that it's okay to feel hungry."

Her words really struck a chord for me, and I remember thinking, "You mean it's *okay* to feel hungry? I don't actually have to *do* anything about it?" The thought was entirely liberating. For so many of us in the Western world, true hunger is never a real consideration. If we feel like eating, so often the source is something *other* than physical hunger.

If you already know that your anticandida diet is well balanced and nutrient dense and yet you still crave more food, try acknowledging the craving in your own mind, then turn your attention to something else. I like to imagine myself actually addressing the craving as if it were an unwanted marketer who showed up at my door or called me while I was relaxing after dinner. In my head, I respond with something like, "Thanks for that piece of information. Now bug off," as I get back to the task at hand.

8. Meditate on It

In her book *The Willpower Instinct*, Kelly McGonigal notes that one of the easiest and quickest ways to increase willpower is through meditation. As she points out, meditation teaches the brain to be more observant in the moment, ultimately leading to better control of what she calls "won't" power, or the ability to say no to actions that may feel compelling. In addition, she notes, meditation increases blood flow to the brain's prefrontal cortex, which is where our self-control is housed.

Another useful aspect of meditation is its relation to heart rate variability, or healthy variations in heart rate that occur all the time (as opposed to arrhythmias, which are unhealthy variations). While stress and anxiety decrease the healthy form of heart rate variability, meditation also helps restore the healthy kind. And interestingly, people with better heart rate variability are also able to resist temptations of all kinds—including food cravings—better than those without it. As McGonigal puts it, "Stress is the enemy of self-control."[2]

9. Sleep on It

Another factor to consider while on the diet (and beyond) is how much sleep you get each night. McGonigal also mentions that on average, most North Americans nowadays get two hours less sleep per night than people did in 1960. That lack of sleep can create problems with impulse control (e.g., willpower to resist foods we crave). So it's well worth trying to get a full night's sleep each night as well. For most people, the most beneficial amount is seven to eight hours per night.

10. Go Back to the Future

Finally, remember that the anticandida diet is something you do for yourself, to improve the quality of your life and your future. When a craving hits, it's useful to contemplate why you took on this challenge in the first place. Ultimately, you want to feel better and gain control of the habits (food-related or otherwise) that triggered the candida. When you feel like eating something that will thwart that goal, keep your eye on the prize: a healthier body and mind down the road!

Challenge 4: Time Constraints

Everyone is pressed for time in our society. And one of the major worries about going on the ACD is that it will consume most of the day to cook everything from scratch, made worse by the fact that most people on the diet are already feeling weak and time-strapped.

While it's true that some of the recipes may require a bit of planning, I offer several time-saving techniques to cut back on preparation and cooking time. Look for tips in Chapter 5.

Different recipes require varying amounts of prep time, from really quick to longer, weekend-appropriate recipes. You can stick entirely with the quick ones if they work better for you, or engage in a Sunday cook-a-thon and then freeze enough for later. (To help you decide which recipes work best for you, I've coded those that are easy to make. Recipes with this icon (Q&E) can be whipped up in thirty minutes or less).

Challenge 5: Social Situations

When I first explain to people what "anticandida diet" means, their reaction is inevitably one of either shock ("How can you live without Starbucks?") or pity ("I'm so sorry to hear that"). They may end by patting me on the shoulder with a "poor you" look in their eyes. But this emotional reaction is entirely misplaced.

Contrary to popular belief, I do still attend birthday parties, work events, holiday celebrations, weddings, and other social occasions and I no longer worry (too much) about what to eat when traveling. (Oh, and I don't do without Starbucks; I just order a green or herbal tea instead.) And it can be the same for you. See Chapter 14 for how to navigate social situations and eating outside the home with aplomb.

Part II

The ACD Kitchen:
Ingredients and Recipes

CHAPTER 5

In the Kitchen: Your ACD Pantry and Ingredient Substitutions

Now comes the fun part: the food! Stocking your pantry exclusively with foods that are both nutrient packed and don't contribute to problems with candida will ensure you always have good choices on hand and are therefore much (much) less likely to stray from the diet.

I know that some of these ingredients will be new to many of you; when I first started the ACD, they were new to me, too. And while learning to use new ingredients may take a little time, as you continue to follow the diet and prepare recipes with these newfangled anticandida foods, I promise that soon they'll feel totally familiar and you'll come to love them as much as all the staples you likely have on hand right now. Whipped cream (from coconut milk) is perhaps one of the most delectable, indulgent tasting foods on earth—I absolutely adore ice cream made from it, more than I ever did dairy ice cream. And I have no doubt you'll develop a hankering for fresh greens in no time once you taste the As-You-Like Kale Salad (page 172). Until then and while you're still learning, it's a good idea to start with the essentials, expanding your repertoire as you go along. Here are some of the "must-have" ingredients I'd suggest buying when you first start out.

Basic Anticandida Diet Pantry List

Chia seeds: These tiny, gray, pearl-like seeds are a nutrition powerhouse, with more omega-3s and protein than flaxseeds (and unlike flax, they don't need to be ground up to impart their health benefits). Eat them whole on salads or side dishes, add to smoothies (they'll thicken up considerably), or use as an egg substitute. One of my favorite breakfasts is Basic Chia Pudding (page 101).

Flours: Coconut flour, chickpea flour, and carob flour are great choices to get you started. Anywhere you see Garfava flour (a mixture of garbanzo [chickpea] and fava bean flour) in my recipes, you can safely substitute chickpea. I really like the slightly milder flavor of Garfava flour, so do give it a try, if you can find it, as you go along on the diet (see Resources, page 242). Carob is rarely used on its own as a flour but more often replaces cocoa in sweet treats (and while it doesn't actually taste like chocolate, I do love its unique, slightly sweet, and slightly nutty flavor).

As a general rule, I advocate avoiding store-bought grain-based flours in early stages of the diet (see Chapter 4), but as you move to later stages and begin to reintroduce flours, you can aim for buckwheat, quinoa, and millet flours as staples.

Fruits: The only fruits permitted in Stage 1 are lime, lemon, avocado, and cranberries. You can usually find whole unsweetened cranberries in the frozen food section, even when they're out of season. In the months leading up to Christmas, I tend to buy bags of fresh cranberries and keep them in my freezer until I need them. That way, I have access to cranberries all year round.

Grains and pseudo-grains: Most grains are verboten in the early stages of the diet, but I do love quinoa and buckwheat (if you're not a fan of the latter, you can usually substitute quinoa) and, of course, brown rice (I use brown basmati for faster cooking). If you've never had millet before, it's also a great grain to try, with a mild flavor and texture much like those of quinoa. And here's a bonus with millet: it's the only grain that's considered to be more alkaline than acidic. Once you're familiar with these, and after Stage 2, you can add teff, amaranth, and (farther down the road) steel-cut oats, if you can tolerate them.

Healthy oils: The very best oil you can use for any application is organic coconut oil, not only because it can withstand heat without degradation, but also because it contains caprylic acid, a natural antifungal. Extra-virgin olive oil is another good choice, as is sesame oil in small quantities. Start with coconut and olive, and expand from there.

Herbs and seasonings: As much as possible, aim to use fresh herbs in your cooking. For these recipes, you can start out with fresh parsley, cilantro, and basil to great effect. I also love fresh dill in soups and salads. Basic dried herbs and seasonings for the diet include dried oregano, basil, parsley, sea salt (aim for one that has some color, either gray or pink, as it will contain more minerals), freshly ground black pepper, curry powder, ground cumin, cayenne pepper, and smoked paprika.

To replace your wheat- and sugar-laden soy sauce, choose Bragg Liquid Aminos (a fermented seasoning made from soybeans alone) or wheat-free tamari (a naturally fermented form of soy sauce). For those allergic to soy, coconut aminos are a newcomer to the market, with a slightly more "fermented" flavor than traditional soy sauce. All three can be found in health food stores or some natural foods sections of your local supermarket.

Lacto-fermented sauerkraut or kimchi: Lacto-fermented sauerkraut and kimchi (a Korean spicy sauerkraut) are filled with live bacteria because they're fermented naturally, without using vinegar. As a result, these foods must also be refrigerated from the moment they're ready to eat, and you'll find them in the refrigerator section of your supermarket or health food store.

Leafy greens: These include kale, romaine lettuce, spinach, baby greens, Swiss chard. Opt for darker varieties and, if you like them, bitter greens (dandelion, arugula, collards, rapini, etc.) as they help stimulate bile production and make life easier for your liver, the major detoxification organ in the body.

Miso: Miso is another naturally fermented soy product used in Japanese cuisine. This thick, flavorful, spreadlike substance is meant to be used sparingly as a condiment. Miso is very salty, and a little goes a long way. The darker the color, the more intense the flavor, so I tend toward "white" or "mellow" miso (white or yellow). You can find miso in Asian groceries or the refrigerated section of your health food store. Miso will keep almost indefinitely in the refrigerator.

Nuts and seeds: We talked about chia seeds earlier in this list; additional must-haves include dried unsweetened shredded coconut, raw almonds, raw walnuts, raw pumpkin seeds, raw hemp seeds, raw sesame seeds, and raw flaxseeds. Apart from the healthy oils, fiber, and protein they contain, most of these can be used to make homemade milks, so you'll want to have them on hand.

Nut and seed butters: Again, almond tops the list, but other nut (or seed) butters are useful in many recipes. I also use coconut butter for many of the desserts (see page 100 to learn how to make your own—much more economical!). If you buy prepared nut butters, they should be unsweetened and contain only one ingredient: whatever nut or seed from which they're made (or, at most, added salt). Avoid nut and seed butters with added oils; these oils are usually highly processed and not healthy.

Nondairy milks: In the early stages of the diet, I'd highly recommend steering clear of alternative milks that come in a carton. These products tend to contain all manner of processed fillers and other ingredients that could put a strain on the immune system and hijack your healing (I do sometimes use them now that I'm in a maintenance stage of the diet, but always make sure they contain no added sweeteners and as few ingredients as possible). Best choices are almond, coconut, flax, or hemp. Rice milk is delicious, but it is quite high in natural sugars, so not the best choice for someone beginning an anticandida diet. You'll also find easy recipes for homemade nut and seed milks in Chapter 6.

Other beverages: For variety, I'd suggest buying a few favorite herbal teas and green tea (excluding jasmine); you can also drink unsweetened 100 percent cranberry juice (just dilute with about four times as much water for a glass of juice, and sweeten with stevia to taste, if you like).

Raw cacao powder: Raw cacao is a great healthier substitute for unsweetened cocoa powder when you are craving something chocolate. It's not as acidic as regular cocoa, and it digests more easily. Like cocoa, though, raw cacao powder does contain some caffeine, and it can trigger cravings in some people. If you find it does that for you, wait a month or two before introducing it (and use carob powder as a substitute in the meantime).

Root vegetables: At a minimum, you'll want to stock carrots, sweet potato, beets, and rutabaga.

Sea vegetables: Another term for "seaweed," sea vegetables include the gamut of nourishing plants from the sea, such as nori (the square sheets used to wrap sushi), arame, wakame, dulse, and others. If you're new to sea vegetables and not sure you'd like them, start with either nori sheets (see recipe for Raw Sushi with Spicy Ginger-Miso Sauce, page 183) or arame, which are both fairly mild. (The Veggie Fried Quinoa [or Rice] with Arame and Edamame, page 195, is a nice starting point.)

Other staples: For many recipes in this book, psyllium husks are an essential ingredient. The whole husks can be purchased in most health food stores. As a source of (flavorless) fiber, psyllium husks also act as a binder for gluten-free vegan baked goods. In addition, psyllium works as a kind of "brush" to help sweep away toxins from the digestive tract along with stool. Psyllium is a wonderful addition to any anticandida regime. Some recipes also call for baking soda, baking powder (be sure it's aluminum-free and gluten-free), vanilla powder (used to replace vanilla if you can't find alcohol-free extract), and protein powders (hemp or pea/bean are the best choices—look for brands that are made of just hemp or pea protein without fillers).

Sweeteners: You'll definitely want to invest in some pure stevia extract, either liquid or powdered. When you're craving something sweet, stevia is still, in my opinion, the best way to meet that craving without sacrificing your progress on the diet or triggering more cravings. Of all the low-glycemic sweeteners, stevia is the one I use daily. My two favorite brands are NuNaturals and SweetLeaf.

Other zero-glycemic sweeteners are yacon syrup (a dark, sticky syrup that resembles molasses) and lo han guo (monkfruit), available as a liquid or powder as well. Once you're into Stage 2, look for lucuma, a low-glycemic fruit native to South America. The dehydrated fruit is sold as a powder that can be used to sweeten or flavor baked goods or other treats. I find that its flavor is akin to butterscotch or caramel and use it sometimes in desserts.

Tempeh: This cousin to tofu is made from fermented soybeans (and sometimes other beans or grains) and has a nutty, rich taste. Like tofu, it soaks up marinades very well. It can usually be found refrigerated or frozen in the health food store (more mainstream groceries are carrying tempeh, too). Use tempeh as you would tofu, or crumble and use instead of ground meat. Note that tempeh should not be eaten raw; always steam or bake first.

ACD Ingredient Substitutions

As you continue with the diet, you'll come to learn which foods you can easily re-create in an "ACD-friendly" version and which you can't. For the most part, I've been able to revamp almost every recipe I've attempted simply by substituting more natural, whole food ingredients for those that are processed, or contain sugar or alcohol.

To best determine how to substitute for conventional ingredients, first examine a few factors relating to each ingredient:

What kind of food is it? Is it a vegetable or fruit? a root vegetable vs. leafy green or other? a beverage? a protein, starch, fat . . . and so on? Your substitute should fall into the same category, or else exhibit qualities that are very similar to foods in that category.

What does it taste like? Is it sweet, sour, salty, bitter, or umami (savory)? Look for a substitute with a similar taste profile.

What texture does it contribute to the final product? Think about how the food is once cooked or mixed with the other ingredients: is it a thickener? Is it granular? chewy? crunchy? sticky? . . . and so on. Aim to reproduce that texture in your final product, too. For example, when you substitute a gluten-free flour for a non-gluten-free one (e.g., chickpea flour for all-purpose flour), you may need to add some kind of binder to account for the gluten. You'll also need to add something to lighten up the final product, as non-gluten-free baked goods are fluffier than gluten-free ones.

How much of the ingredient do you need? Consider whether your replacement food should be used in the same amount as the original, less, or more?

Foods That Can Be Used as Substitutes

Flour

What to use for:

Flour in baking: As mentioned earlier, when you first start the diet, it's not advisable to use purchased flours because they can be highly processed. However, it's really easy to make your own "flours" by grinding whole grains. Such recipes as Fluffy Pancakes (page 120) and Sunday Night Roast (page 196) use this method.

Chickpea (or other bean/legume) flour, ground nuts, and ground seeds all make suitable substitutes for flour in baked goods.

Flour as a thickener: I've found that chickpea or other legume flours work well as thickeners in sauces or gravies (see Perfect Golden Gravy, page 177).

Instead of pasta, use: Herbed Grain-Free Gnocchi (page 188); spiralized or grated zucchini, carrot, daikon radish, or sweet potato.

Sweeteners

Instead of sugar, use:

Stevia: When you first start out, stevia will be your go-to sweetener. If you've never used stevia before, here are some key points to get you started:

- *Less is more.* This is my mantra when it comes to stevia. Keep in mind that, in some cases (depending on the brand you use), stevia can be up to one hundred times sweeter than sugar. You don't need very much at all! And since some people report a slightly bitter or metallic aftertaste where stevia is concerned, I've found that using the bare minimum required to achieve an acceptable level of sweetness (which may be less sweet than you're used to) is the way to avoid any bitterness. If you learn to love things less sweet, eventually they will also taste very sweet to you!

- *Liquid or powder can be used interchangeably in a ratio of 2:1.* In other words, if a recipe calls for ¼ teaspoon (1 ml) of powder, you can use ½ teaspoon (2.5 ml) of liquid instead. Around 20 drops equals ¼ teaspoon (1 ml).

- *Stevia works best combined with other sweet flavors.* Once you're further into the diet, you can combine it with yacon syrup, coconut sugar, or coconut nectar (most of my baked goods use this trick to great effect—no one realizes they contain stevia at all). In savory dishes, use it in dressings, to sweeten tea, on breakfast cereal, and so on.

- *Be careful with chocolate + stevia combos.* Many people report that, used in combination, stevia and chocolate can bring out the bitterness in each other. I always aim for the minimum sweetness required when sweetening chocolate this way, to avoid an aftertaste. Replacing part of the cacao with carob powder in recipes can also help mitigate any bitterness.

Coconut sugar: Once you're into Stage 3 of the diet, coconut sugar is a fabulous go-to dry sweetener. As a rule, I use about half as much sugar as called for in a recipe, topping up the sweetness levels with stevia as a way to keep the overall glycemic load of the recipe as low as possible.

Coconut nectar: Although it's a thick, sticky liquid, coconut nectar can also be used in place of sugar in recipes in Stage 3 and beyond. Use three quarters of the original amount of liquid in the recipe if you opt to replace sugar with coconut nectar. I also usually combine coconut nectar with stevia when I use it.

Fruit and vegetable purees: Once you're able to incorporate some fruits back into your diet in Stage 2 or later, you can add homemade (sugar-free) applesauce or fresh pear puree to foods to boost the sweetness levels. Similarly, sweet potato puree is a great way to increase the sweetness level of baked goods, such as pancakes, muffins, or desserts (I use it in the Grain-Free Fudgy Brownies, for instance, on page 206).

Carob: Although carob isn't a sweetener on its own, using carob powder in place of some (or all) the cocoa in a recipe will render it slightly sweeter and less bitter.

Cinnamon: On its own, ground cinnamon's taste is slightly sweet. Added to baked goods or roasted vegetables, it does confer a slight sweetness to recipes as well.

Instead of molasses, use:

Yacon syrup: Thick, sticky and dark like molasses, yacon is the syrup from a tuberous root that grows in the Andes Mountains. To my palate, yacon tastes like what I imagine molasses would taste like if it were fermented, with a slightly tangy flavor. With an extremely low glycemic index (some sources cite it as low as zero), yacon makes a good addition when you're seeking a molasses flavor or in foods that are already fairly robust. I always use yacon in conjunction with another sweetener.

Eggs

Apart from meringue or soufflé, it's really not difficult to replace eggs in your cooking. If you've got favorite old recipes that you'd like to revamp for the ACD, here are some common egg replacements. (Note that all my recipes are already formulated without eggs, so there's no need to add or subtract anything from them.)

Each of the following works well in place of one egg in baked goods. When using in baked goods (e.g., biscuits or pancakes), it's best to replace no more than two eggs in any one recipe.

Instead of eggs, use:

Ground flax: Flax is my favorite egg substitute for baked goods. Each time you wish to replace an egg in a recipe, combine 1 tablespoon (15 ml) of finely ground flaxseeds (also known as flaxseed meal) with 3 tablespoons (45 ml) of water in a small bowl; allow to sit for three to five minutes, until thick and jelled. (I use flax this way in the Fluffy Pancakes recipe, page 120.)

Ground chia: Like flax, chia transforms into a viscous, slightly gluey substance when mixed with water, perfect to use as an egg substitute. Because ground chia absorbs so much more liquid than flax, however, I've always found that I need only about half the chia compared to flax to achieve the same results. For each egg, use 2 teaspoons (10 ml) of chia and 3 tablespoons (45 ml) of water; allow to sit until jelled, then add to your recipes.

Avocado: Because of its high fat content, avocado makes an awesome egg substitute in baked goods! Use about ¼ cup (60 ml) of avocado puree in place of one egg. When baked, the color turns slightly yellow (not green), so be careful when choosing this option (I like to use it in chocolate-based, or darker, baked goods for that reason).

Sweet potato puree: If you haven't guessed yet, I adore sweet potatoes. Adding them as an additional binder in baked goods is just one more great use for this marvelous vegetable. As with fruit purees, use about ¼ cup (60 ml) of sweet potato puree for each egg you replace.

Cream/Dairy

A simple and easy substitute for milk in all recipes is any kind of unsweetened alternative milk, such as almond, hemp, or coconut (see how to make your own on pages 97, 98, and 99). As you'll see in the recipe chapters as well, coconut "cream" makes a great substitute for dairy cream (and I've even come to love the flavor more than that of dairy cream).

Gluten/Binders

Since all my recipes are gluten-free, my recipes also require some kind of binding agent that can replace the gluten. Most gluten-free bakers use either xanthan or guar gum; a newcomer in this category is also psyllium husk.

You'll notice that most of my recipes with psyllium also include one or more of the items from the "eggs" list (page 85). Over many years of trial and error, I've found that using a single ingredient to replace the binding power of both eggs and gluten is often insufficient, but two mixed together works like a charm. I tend to think of one as an egg substitute and the other as a gluten substitute.

Psyllium husk: A recent addition to the gluten-free baker's arsenal, psyllium husk has been around for quite some time as a treatment for constipation (that's right, it's the main ingredient in Metamucil). Psyllium husks are a form of tasteless fiber that adds binding power to your baked goods. Depending on the recipe, I'll use anywhere from 1 tablespoon (15 ml) to ¼ cup (60 ml) of psyllium in my baked goods.

Xanthan or guar gum: These gums are the most common replacements for gluten in baked goods and can usually be used interchangeably (though xanthan is more stable in baked goods, and guar gum loses its sticking power when added to a highly acidic mixture). Xanthan gum is often made from corn, so if you have a corn allergy, be sure to use Bob's Red Mill or Namaste brands, which are (at the time of this writing) both corn-free.[1,2]

White Wine (in cooking)

Because I've only ever been a social drinker, giving up a glass of wine when out to dinner or socializing with friends wasn't really a problem for me; I'm just as happy with some sparkling water or a fizzy ACD-Friendly Fruity Sipper (page 116). As I began to revamp some of my older recipes to render them ACD-friendly, however, I realized that many contained wine, so I needed a substitute.

Recipes using white wine often rely on both the acid and the tannins in the wine to help enhance flavors and also create a tender final product. Because my dishes are all vegan, there are no worries about tenderizing, so lemon juice makes a great substitute to offer a similar acidic flavor. If you're subbing for a sweet white wine, use stevia to enhance the sweetness. For each cup of wine, I use about ¼ cup (60 ml) of lemon juice plus ¾ cup (180 ml) of water, and stevia to taste. Another useful substitute for white wine is raw apple cider vinegar, about 2 tablespoons (30 ml) added to 1 cup (240 ml) of water.

Red Wine (in cooking)

Because red wine has a more robust, less sweet flavor and contains more tannins than white wine, recipes that call for it require something equally bold as a replacement. Unsweetened cranberry juice is a great source of tannins as well, and the color resembles that of red wine in the final product (as in the Tempeh "Bourguignon," page 198). With cranberry juice, be sure to add a touch of stevia to cut the sourness. I generally use about ½ cup (120 ml) of 100 percent cranberry juice (undiluted) with ½ cup (120 ml) of water for each cup of red wine in a recipe. You can also try dark, red herbal teas, such as Red Zinger, instead of the juice.

Applesauce

Many vegan or oil-free recipes call for applesauce as an egg replacer or binder, but, when you first begin the ACD, fruit is often not allowed at all. In those cases, I've found that pureed spaghetti squash makes a great substitute (add stevia to taste). When blended, the squash has just the right balance of moisture and body to approximate the same results as applesauce. If you can't find spaghetti squash where you are, yellow summer squash also works (or use zucchini and peel it first to avoid adding a green tint to your baked goods).

Bananas

I never realized how many recipes—from smoothies to vegan soft-serve "ice cream" to baked goods—call for bananas until I was no longer able to eat them. I've found that, in most cases, an equal amount of pear puree can be used instead of mashed banana or frozen banana in any of these recipes. I use it in the Classic Green Smoothie (page 113) as well as the Vanilla Ice Cream (page 220) in this way. (Note that pear isn't permitted in early stages of the diet, though.)

Dates

Even once you've gone through the stages of the diet and move to Stage 3, you may still find that dates are too sweet for you (I've been able to consume them on rare occasions, but too much can still trigger a reaction for me). On the other hand, prunes are equally dark, almost as sweet, and sticky and make a perfect replacement for dates in baked goods or other sweet dishes. They're also much lower on the glycemic index than dates (approximately 29 vs. 62,[3] respectively). I usually add a bit of stevia to recipes using prunes, to amp up the sweetness that dates would impart.

Raisins

Like dates, raisins are usually too sweet for someone on a candida diet—even a maintenance diet—to eat in any quantity. Where raisins are normally called for, I tend to use either chopped prunes, goji berries, or golden berries. Goji berries, a small, oval, red, dried superfood fruit originating in Tibet, are now widely available in most health food stores or the natural foods section of most major supermarkets. They are known to have a high ORAC value (a measure of the amount of antioxidant power in foods) and a low glycemic index. Golden berries, also known as "Incan berries," are round, darkly golden antioxidant-rich berries from the Andes Mountains, with a texture much like raisins and tart, tangy-sweet flavor. Some people find their flavor too intense, but I love them. I use them regularly as replacements for raisins as well. Both goji berries and golden berries should be reserved for later stages of the diet, however.

Chocolate

As someone who grew up on milk chocolate and considered it my favorite food, I was resistant to the idea that I'd never again consume it after being on the ACD. I do still miss the flavor of milk chocolate, but, knowing how unhealthy it is and how the ingredients are often derived, I know I'd never *want* to eat it again even if I could. Now, organic, healthy, homemade chocolate? Well, that's another story! You'll find a Homemade Chocolate recipe on page 205. It can be converted to chips or chunks but unfortunately doesn't work in baked goods as the oil melts too much. If you're willing to splurge on pure cacao butter, use that instead of the coconut oil and your chocolate will hold its shape at room temperature, or in baked goods.

Mushrooms

Because they are a fungus, common mushrooms are normally excluded from the anti-candida diet (for info on keeping mold at bay, see page 89). If they're a main ingredient in a recipe (e.g., sautéed mushrooms over a burger or slice of Sunday Night Roast, page 196), then no, you likely won't be able to substitute for them. But I've found that most recipes calling for mushrooms really just require something earthy and umami, with a high water content. The best veggie sub I've discovered in most cases is chopped eggplant. When cooked, its color darkens, and it also offers a robust, slightly umami taste. Depending on the recipe, black beans can also work in place of mushrooms.

Yeast

Obviously, yeast isn't an option on an antiyeast diet. How, then, to make your baked goods rise? Generally, anticandida breads and other baked goods rely on chemical leaveners, such as baking powder and baking soda, to acquire the airiness of traditional baked goods. Note that gluten-free baking also requires a bit of an extra "lift" as they don't naturally rise as much as non-gluten-free ones. I like to use a mixture of baking powder, baking soda, and raw apple cider vinegar in my baked goods. Double-acting baking powder (most brands today) is designed to begin rising as soon as the wet ingredients are added, then again when the item is placed in the warm oven; and baking soda combined with raw apple cider vinegar creates a chemical reaction that increases the leavening. Just take care not to overmix baked goods leavened this way, as their structure is often delicate and it's all too easy to stir out any of the air bubbles that are essential for light baked goods.

Peanuts

Almond butter makes a great (and delicious) substitute in most recipes (see the Asian Napa Cabbage Salad dressing, for instance, on page 168), but it's thinner than peanut butter for spreading. In that case, I often use homemade nut butters, which are naturally thicker and hold their shape better (see recipes on page 99). Many people find that cashew or sunflower seed butter tastes very much like peanut butter as well.

Keep Mold at Bay in Your Pantry

It goes without saying that avoiding all foods that are made from, or contain, mold or fungus will help prevent a relapse of candida symptoms. While some sources suggest that moldy foods have no connection to candida,[4] others claim that, because molds belong in the same kingdom of life (the fungal kingdom) as candida, the body may react in a similar fashion to both and mount an immune response to any fungi. At the very least, molds, whether in the home and on foods, produce mycotoxins that tax the immune system, something you should avoid when your system has already been stressed to the max by a bout of candida overgrowth.

Foods Most Likely to Harbor Mold

Although most foods can become a breeding ground for mold, certain items tend to harbor more mold than others. According to *The Fungus Link* by Dr. David Holland and Doug Kaufmann,[5] the top ten moldy foods in descending order are:

- Alcoholic beverages (especially those made from grains or fruit)
- Corn
- Wheat (and most products made from wheat, e.g., bread, crackers, cookies, cakes, muffins)
- Barley
- Sugar cane and sugar beets
- Sorghum
- Peanuts
- Rye
- Cottonseed (often used in animal feed)
- Hard cheeses (especially any with mold already in them, such as blue cheese)
- Other foods known to harbor mold are dried fruits (raisins, prunes, dried apricots, etc.); most tomato products; beer, wine, and wine vinegars; processed meats (hot dogs, salami, bologna, etc.); hamburger; overripe fruits and vegetables; and any product of aspergillus fermentation (includes regular soy sauces, conventional chocolate, black teas, fruit juices, and others).[6]

To prevent mold from growing on foods that you've prepared yourself, freeze any leftovers (this will slow down mold growth), and don't leave cooked foods at room temperature for more than two hours.

Preventing Mold on Fresh Produce

Some fruits and vegetables ripen more fully at room temperature and just taste better that way. Others (e.g., apples) retain their crispness or juiciness longer in the refrigerator. Beware whichever you choose, though: fresh produce (especially if it's organic) can quickly harbor mold—without any outward signs, so we won't know until it's too late.

While I loved every aspect of my time in nutrition school, one of the lessons that struck me (perhaps "haunted" is a better term) was our cellular biology segment on molds. Molds grow by extending hyphae (rootlike filaments) to feed on dead organic matter; they grow below the surface to digest and absorb nutrients; then, at maturity, a fuzzy growth called a fruiting body appears on the outside surface (that's the green fuzz we notice on our fruit or vegetables).

By the time the fruiting body is visible, mold has already infiltrated the inside of that fruit or vegetable. In other words, simply cutting off any exterior mold from a piece of fresh produce or cheese is not enough to rid it of mold; by the time you can see the mold, there will always be more of it inside that you cannot see. When faced with a moldy orange, I now always throw it away rather than try to salvage the "other half"; in fact, if the moldy section was touching any other food directly, even if that food still "looks" good, I throw that one away, too.

To prevent mold from growing on produce before you ingest it, always wash your fresh produce in a solution of water and either raw apple cider vinegar or grapefruit seed extract. According to the late Dr. Vincent Marinkovich, an immunologist who devoted his life to battling diseases related to mold, washing fruits and vegetables in a solution of ten drops of grapefruit seed extract in a sinkful of fresh water will destroy any molds on the food. Similarly, boiling root vegetables (e.g., potatoes or carrots) in a solution of water and a teaspoon (5 ml) of Ester-C powder (a form of vitamin C) can eliminate many mycotoxins on the vegetables as well.[7]

TIPS FOR RECIPE SUCCESS

Cooking with new ingredients, especially if you're not accustomed to using whole foods, can be a learning curve. Here are some of my best tips to ensure that you have success in the kitchen and spend as little time as possible chopping, mixing, stirring, or cooking!

For additional convenience, the recipes that take less than thirty minutes have been marked with ⓆⓊⒺ.

Before You Cook

1. *Shop with a list.* Using a list will help streamline the time you spend in the grocery store; it will also help prevent impulse purchases of ingredients not on the ACD.

2. *Handle food only as many times as you absolutely must.* There's an efficiency tip in business that uses the acronym "OHIO": only handle it once. In other words, if you open an e-mail, read it and act on it immediately instead of leaving it in your inbox and having to go back to it later.

I try to apply the same rule to my groceries: If I bring home lettuce or leafy greens, I wash, spin, and store them as soon as I get home so that they're placed in the refrigerator ready to go into my recipes. That way, I save time when I'm cooking as I don't have to open, trim, wash, and spin them at that time. Cleaned and dried leafy greens will keep for up to a week if stored in a covered container, lined with clean paper toweling, in the refrigerator. In the same way, you can trim, peel, and store carrots or celery in water for immediate use.

When You're Ready to Cook

1. *Read the entire recipe first.* You'll avoid any surprise steps this way (e.g., having to soak dried legumes or preheating an oven) and ensure you understand the instructions.

2. *Set out ingredients and materials in advance.* Known among chefs as *mise en place*, the technique of gathering all the ingredients before you start to cook and preparing any that may need some time (e.g., chopped onions or garlic, or melted coconut oil) will actually speed the process overall. When you prep your *mise en place*, you should also grease pans or line cookie sheets, pull the processor out of the cupboard, and so on.

3. *Cook in bulk (and the freezer is your friend!).* Once a week, I prepare a huge batch of two to four types of grains and legumes that I'll use throughout the rest of the week. I portion them into 2 cup (500 ml) containers and freeze for later use. I also try to cook batches of Glazed Tempeh (page 111) and any dressings or sauces that I know I'll be using later, to store in the fridge. You can bake Grain-Free Sandwich Bread (page 102), even cook up Fluffy Pancakes (page 120) or ACD Whole-Grain Waffles (page 119) in advance and freeze for later use.

After You Cook

1. Wrap and store food as quickly as possible; freeze everything you can. Label with the name of the dish, number of servings, and date frozen.

2. Package food in single servings for easy access and use.

A NOTE ABOUT STAGES

The stages noted in recipes pertain to the basic version of the diet. If you are on the "Fast Track" diet, be sure to avoid any recipes with grains, legumes, or starchy vegetables, even if they are labeled "Good for: all stages."

CHAPTER 6

Cooking Basics and Staple Recipes

The following chapters provide recipes for a wide array of meals, from smoothies to snacks and, yes, even desserts. This chapter focuses on some basic cooking strategies I've mentioned earlier (soaking, sprouting) as well as making your own basics, from nut butters and milks to condiments.

Soaking Nuts or Seeds

Almost all the nut or seed milk recipes in this book call for soaked nuts or seeds, as this reduces the enzyme inhibitors and renders them much easier to digest.

Soaking your nuts and seeds couldn't be easier. Simply choose a clean glass jar that holds at least twice the volume of nuts or seeds you wish to use (so, for 1 cup [180 g] of raw almonds, for instance, choose a jar with a total volume of at least 2 cups [500 ml]). Place the nuts or seeds in the jar and fill with filtered water to cover; loosely cover with the jar lid. Allow to sit at room temperature anywhere from 8 to 12 hours, then rinse and store in fresh water, covered, in the refrigerator; use within one day for nut/seed milk, raw pâté, and so on. If you do continue to soak them, some will eventually form tiny sprouts on one end; this is fine (but never store soaked nuts longer than 1 week, in any case).

Soaking Grains or Legumes

Like nuts and seeds, grains and legumes become more digestible after being soaked or sprouted, which removes some enzyme inhibitors and reduces the phytic acid that can prevent our digestive systems from effectively absorbing nutrients. For those that will be cooked (grains and most legumes), simply soak as you would nuts or seeds, then drain and rinse before cooking. Grains and legumes that benefit most from soaking include rice, quinoa, millet, amaranth, whole oat groats, black beans, kidney beans, white (e.g., great northern) beans, lima beans, dried fava beans, pinto beans, black-eyed peas, romano (a.k.a. borlotti or cranberry) beans, or lentils.

Sprouting Legumes or Seeds

To sprout legumes or seeds (to eat raw), you'll need a bit of equipment: mason jars with lids (or an elastic band that fits snugly over the jar), cheesecloth or fine mesh (cut to fit over the top of the jar with about 1 inch [2.5 cm] excess). The whole process will take 2 to 3 days.

Begin by placing about a tablespoon of legumes or seeds in the bottom of the jar and filling with room-temperature water; allow to soak at room temperature for 8 to 12 hours. With the cheesecloth secured over the top of the jar, screw on the original canning lid (remove the solid insert so that the cloth is exposed in the middle), or, if using mesh, secure it with the elastic. Pour out the water through the covering and place the jar upside down on an angle in the draining rack of your sink or upside down in a small bowl.

Rinse the legumes or seeds twice a day (morning and evening) by pouring fresh water through the covering into the jar, swirling the contents around, and then carefully draining through the covering. Place the jar back into the rack or bowl each time.

After about 48 hours, you should begin to see tiny sprouts (it may take up to 3 days, depending on the legume or seed). Once the sprout "tails" are about ¼ inch (6 mm) long, they're ready to eat, though you can allow them to grow twice as long if you wish. Once they're ready, rinse and drain well, then store in a covered container in the refrigerator for up to 3 days. My favorite sprouts to prepare this way are mung beans, chickpeas (garbanzo beans), brown lentils, whole peas, fennel seeds, and broccoli seeds. Most legumes and seeds will sprout this way, but note that they must be truly raw to sprout (flax and chia seeds are the exception; they won't sprout and can be used either dry or soaked).

Dehydrating Nuts or Seeds

After you've soaked your nuts or seeds, you may wish to dehydrate them rather than keep them in water in the refrigerator. Dehydrating allows you to preserve the benefits of raw nuts and seeds while converting them to a form that can keep almost indefinitely at room temperature. To dehydrate soaked nuts or seeds, simply drain very well, then spread out in a single layer on a dehydrator sheet and dehydrate at 115°F (46°C) for 8 to 12 hours, until dry and crispy. Use as you would toasted nuts or seeds.

Basic Nut or Seed Milk
Good for: all stages

Store-bought nut and seed milks are certainly convenient, but it's easy to make them at home, too—they are just as tasty (and without any preservatives or added sweeteners, can be much healthier). The hardest part is remembering to soak the nuts! I like creamy milks; if you prefer something a little thinner, add more water before you blend. If you want a seed milk that doesn't require soaking or straining, see Hemp Seed Milk (page 98).

MAKES ABOUT 3 CUPS (720 ML) MILK

1 to 1½ cups (240 to 360 ml) raw nuts or seeds of choice,
   depending on how creamy you want the milk
4 cups (1 L) filtered water
Pinch of fine sea salt (optional)
Stevia (optional)

Soak the nuts (see page 95) in water for 4 to 6 hours. Drain and place in a high-powered blender with the filtered water, then blend for 1 minute until smooth and creamy.

Strain the milk, using a clean cheesecloth or nut milk bag, squeezing out as much of the liquid as possible. Add the salt or stevia to taste, if using. Store the milk in a clean glass jar in the refrigerator for no more than 3 days.

Tip: Straining nut milk can seem tricky at first, but it's quite easy and becomes second nature over time. The easiest way is to purchase a nut milk bag made just for this purpose; it fits neatly over the mouth of your blender jug and allows you to "squeeze" out the milk into a bowl, trapping the pulp inside the bag. Another way is to use clean cheesecloth, but be sure to gather all the edges before squeezing, as the pulp has a tendency to escape! A very fine sieve can be used in a pinch to strain nut or seed milk, but the final product will retain some fiber and may be slightly grainy. Nut pulp is great added to raw pâtés or cooked cereal, or mixed into muffin, waffle, or pancake batter (add 2 to 3 tablespoons [30 to 45 ml]) to any batter to increase the fiber content). Freeze any leftover nut or seed pulp until ready to use.

Q&E

Basic Hemp Seed Milk
Good for: all stages

Hemp milk is one of the easiest alternative milks because it doesn't require straining. The seeds themselves are so small and soft that they blend almost perfectly without much pulp. If you prefer a totally pulp-free milk, you can, of course, still strain it. I love the slightly nutty flavor of hemp milk and use it in smoothies or tea, or over ACD-Friendly Grain-Free Granola (page 123).

MAKES 3 CUPS (720 ML) MILK

½ cup (70 g) raw shelled hemp seeds (hemp hearts)
3 cups (720 ml) filtered water
Pinch of fine sea salt (optional)
5 to 15 drops plain or vanilla pure liquid stevia (optional)

Place the seeds and water in a high-powered blender and blend until the liquid becomes white and creamy and the hemp seeds are completely blended in. Strain through a fine sieve, if desired. Add the salt and/or stevia, if using. Store in a glass jar in the refrigerator for up to 4 days. Shake before using.

Homemade Coconut Milk
Q&E
Good for: all stages

Like hemp milk, homemade coconut milk doesn't require soaking, but it does require straining. This easy milk is rich and creamy, with a white appearance that most resembles that of dairy milk.

MAKES 3 TO 4 CUPS (720 TO 960 ML) MILK

1½ to 2 cups (135 to 190 g) unsweetened shredded (dessicated)
    coconut, depending on how creamy you want the milk
4 cups (960 ml) filtered water
Pinch of fine sea salt
5 to 15 drops plain or vanilla pure liquid stevia (optional)

Place all the ingredients in a high-powered blender and blend until the liquid becomes thick and creamy and no traces of coconut are visible. Strain through a nut milk bag or clean cheese-cloth. Store in a glass jar in the refrigerator for up to 4 days.

Basic Nut or Seed Butter
Q&E
Good for: all stages

I love making my own nut and seed butters at home and rarely buy the prepared kind any more, even when I can find brands with 100 percent pure nuts or seeds. I prefer the texture of homemade, which is thicker than the store-bought, and find it's so much more fun to mix different kinds of nuts together for infinite flavor varieties.

MAKES ABOUT 2 CUPS (500 ML) NUT OR SEED BUTTER

4 cups (1 L) lightly toasted nuts or seeds of choice (do not soak
    first)
2 tablespoons to ¼ cup (30 to 60 ml) extra-virgin coconut oil
¼ teaspoon (1 ml) fine sea salt, or more to taste

Once the toasted nuts are cool, place them in the bowl of a food processor and process until they resemble fine bread crumbs. Scrape down the sides of the bowl and keep processing until the mixture forms a ball and eventually smoothes out to become nut butter. At this point, add 2 tablespoons (30 ml) of the coconut oil and the salt and continue to process until very thin and smooth. Add up to 2 tablespoons (30 ml) of the remaining oil, if desired. (The oil is used to thicken the nut butter when refrigerated so that it's spreadable when cold; if you don't mind a thin nut butter, you can leave it out.) Store in clean jars in the refrigerator for up to 3 weeks.

Note: My favorites are almonds, walnuts, cashews, hazelnuts, sunflower seeds, and pumpkin seeds; sesame and hemp seeds are more difficult to use this way. One delicious combination uses about two parts almonds with one part cashews for a creamier, thicker butter than almond alone. Combining hazelnuts and almonds also works really well. Or try flavoring nut butters by adding cacao powder, lucuma powder, carob powder, peppermint extract, or anything else you can think of.

Homemade Coconut Butter
Good for: all stages

Unlike coconut oil (which is pure fat), coconut butter is a puree of dried coconut meat, resulting in a thick, luscious spread much like a nut butter when soft or gently melted (but quite hard at room temperature). While you can buy prepared coconut butter, it's relatively expensive, so I find it's worth the effort to make my own at home.

MAKES ABOUT 2 CUPS (50 ML) COCONUT BUTTER

5 cups (475 g) finely shredded unsweetened coconut

High-powered blender method (not suitable for regular blenders): Start with 3 cups (285 g) finely shredded unsweetened coconut. Blend the coconut, using the tamper to push the contents toward the blades, until almost liquid, about 30 seconds. Add another 2 cups (190 g) of coconut and continue to blend until the mixture is entirely liquefied, another 30 to 45 seconds.

Scrape into a clean jar and store, covered, at room temperature (it will solidify within a few hours). Will keep for up to 6 months.

Food processor method: Place the entire 5 cups (475 g) of coconut in the bowl of your food processor and process until it resembles a paste, for about 5 minutes. Scrape down the sides and continue to process, scraping the sides frequently, until liquefied, up to 5 more minutes. Note that coconut butter made this way will still be slightly grainy, unlike the butter made in a blender. Scrape into a clean jar and store, covered, at room temperature (it will solidify within a few hours). Will keep for up to 6 months.

Basic Chia Pudding
Good for: all stages

Q&E

Chia pudding reminds me of a slightly firmer version of tapioca pudding. It is a staple in most vegan kitchens because it's an easy, no-cook, make-ahead dish that is full of healthy omega-3s and high in protein, making it equally good for break-fast. Plus, it's delicious! Start with this base recipe and experiment with add-ins (e.g., chopped nuts, cacao nibs, or coconut) to suit your own tastes.

MAKES 2 SERVINGS

¼ cup (60 ml) whole chia seeds
1⅓ cups (320 ml) unsweetened almond, hemp, or other
    alternative milk of choice
1 teaspoon (5 ml) pure vanilla extract (optional)
Pinch of fine sea salt
10 to 20 drops plain or flavored pure liquid stevia, or to taste

Place the chia in a small bowl and add the milk and vanilla. Stir well to try to submerge most of the seeds. Allow to sit for 20 to 30 minutes, stirring once after about 5 minutes to prevent clumping. Stir in the salt and stevia. Stir again before serving. Alternatively, combine all the ingredients in a 2 cup (500 ml) glass jar, shake, cover, and allow to sit overnight in the refrig-erator. Stir again before serving, adding more milk if necessary to achieve the desired texture.

Chocolate or Carob Chia Pudding: Add 2 tablespoons (30 ml) of raw cacao powder or carob powder to the pudding with the other ingredients, and increase the milk to 1½ cups (360 ml).

Lemon Chia Pudding: Add the zest of ½ lemon to the pudding with the other ingredients.

Berry Chia Pudding (Stage 2 and beyond): Using an immersion blender, puree ½ cup (120 ml) of berries of choice. Add with the other ingredients.

Pumpkin Chia Pudding: Use only 1 cup (240 ml) of milk and add ⅓ cup (80 ml) of unsweetened pumpkin puree, 1 teaspoon (5 ml) of ground cinnamon, ½ teaspoon (2.5 ml) of ground ginger, and a pinch of ground cloves with the other ingredients.

Grain-Free Sandwich Bread
Good for: all stages

From now on, you'll never be without when you're craving a slice of bread! It's not the same texture as "real" sandwich bread, but this loaf is breadlike, and it keeps well and slices easily. I bake a loaf, let it cool, then cut it into eight pieces, wrap them individually, and freeze them for later. This bread is great slathered with Homemade Coconut Butter (page 100) or My Favorite Hummus (page 161). But beware: this is not a bread to sample warm from the oven; it will be far too moist inside at that point. It firms up as it cools and is actually best the next day. This recipe was one of the testers' favorites.

MAKES 1 LOAF

Coconut oil, for pan (optional)
⅔ cup (160 ml) spaghetti squash puree (see note)
1½ tablespoons (22.5 ml) raw apple cider vinegar
¾ cup (180 ml) vegetable broth or stock
½ cup (120 ml) smooth natural almond butter, tahini, or
    sunflower butter (see note)

5 drops plain pure liquid stevia (optional; it brings out the
   flavors)
3 tablespoons (45 ml) finely ground flaxseeds
3 tablespoons (45 ml) whole psyllium husks (not powder)
1 cup plus 1 tablespoon (150 g) raw pumpkin seeds
2½ teaspoons (12.5 ml) baking powder
1¼ teaspoons (6 ml) baking soda
¼ to ½ teaspoon (1 to 2.5 ml) fine sea salt
⅔ cup (65 g) chickpea flour

Preheat the oven to 325°F (170°C). Line an 8-inch (20 cm) loaf pan with parchment, or grease with coconut oil.

In a medium-size bowl, whisk together the squash, vinegar, broth, almond butter, and stevia. Set aside.

In the bowl of a food processor, blend the flax, psyllium, pumpkin seeds, baking powder, baking soda, salt, and chickpea flour until the mixture resembles a powder. There should be no pieces of pumpkin seed larger than a bread crumb.

Pour the liquid ingredients over the dry ingredients in the processor and blend *just to* combine; *do not overmix*. The mixture may begin to fizz and expand a bit.

Immediately transfer to the prepared loaf pan and very gently smooth the top. Allow to sit undisturbed for 5 minutes.

After 5 minutes, bake the loaf for 70 to 80 minutes, rotating the pan about halfway through, until a tester inserted in the middle comes out clean and the top is very well browned. Let cool completely before removing from the pan and slicing. May be frozen.

Note: This recipe will work with sunflower seed butter, but the final loaf may turn green because compounds in the seeds react with heat. It doesn't affect the taste or nutritional value but may be a slight deterrent visually (unless you're a six-year-old, that is).

Tip: To bake spaghetti squash, place the whole squash on a parchment-lined cookie sheet in a preheated 400°F (200°C) oven for about an hour, until the skin just begins to brown and a knife can be inserted easily. Remove from the oven and allow to cool completely, then cut in half lengthwise and scoop out all the seeds. Scoop the flesh from the skin and then puree the baked flesh in a food processor or blender until perfectly smooth. Any leftover squash puree can be frozen for up to 6 months.

Grain-Free Pizza Crust
Good for: all stages

This crust is sturdy enough to hold in your hands even when covered in toppings. The key here is to bake the crust enough before adding the topping, then continue to bake until done. This is great with the Broccoli-Lemon Pesto (page 181) or Fresh Spicy Tomato Dressing or Sauce (page 180) as a base for your toppings, but equally good with regular tomato sauce (be sure it's homemade without sugar, though).

MAKES 4 SERVINGS

1½ cups (240 g) raw natural almonds or raw pumpkin seeds
⅓ cup (50 g) coconut flour
¼ cup (25 g) chickpea flour
¼ cup (20 g) whole psyllium husks
2 tablespoons (30 ml) finely ground flaxseeds
½ teaspoon (2.5 ml) garlic salt or powder
¼ to ½ teaspoon (1 to 2.5 ml) fine sea salt, or to taste
1 tablespoon (15 ml) dried basil
1 tablespoon (15 ml) baking powder
I medium-size zucchini with skin, trimmed and cut into chunks
     (8 ounces [250 g])
2 tablespoons (30 ml) raw apple cider vinegar
6 tablespoons (90 ml) vegetable broth or water

Preheat the oven to 400°F (200°C). Line a large cookie sheet with parchment.

In the bowl of a food processor, process the almonds, coconut flour, chickpea flour, psyllium, flax, garlic salt, salt, basil, and baking powder until the mixture resembles fine bread crumbs. Transfer to a bowl.

In the same processor bowl (no need to wash it), combine the zucchini, vinegar, and broth and process until smooth. Return the dry mixture to the processor and blend until you have a soft, sticky dough.

Turn the dough onto the cookie sheet and shape into two small rectangles, each about 10 x 6 inches (25 x 15 cm) and ¼ inch (6 mm) thick. Bake for 20 to 25 minutes, until dry on top and very lightly browned on the bottom.

Remove from the oven and top with pesto or tomato sauce and desired toppings (e.g., sliced onion, black olives, red pepper, broccoli, artichoke hearts). Bake for an additional 25 to 30 minutes, until the toppings are cooked and the crust is brown on the edges and bottom. Serve. May be frozen.

Oven-Dried Cranberries
Good for: all stages

Use these anywhere you'd use raisins or conventional dried cranberries. Because these do retain some moisture, however, they can't be stored at room temperature like the regular kind or they'll develop mold. Keep refrigerated for up to 3 days, or freeze in an airtight container.

MAKES ABOUT 1 CUP (240 ML) DRIED CRANBERRIES

2 teaspoons (10 ml) extra-virgin olive oil or melted coconut oil,
   preferably organic
20 drops plain or vanilla pure liquid stevia
12 ounces (340 g) fresh or frozen cranberries, rinsed

Preheat the oven to 225°F (105°C). Line a large, rimmed cookie sheet with parchment.

In the bottom of a large bowl, whisk together the oil and stevia. Add the berries and toss well to coat them all as much as possible. Spread the mixture evenly on the prepared cookie sheet, taking care that the berries are in a single layer and don't overlap.

Bake for 45 minutes, then check. The berries will puff up and then begin to wrinkle like raisins. If necessary, continue to bake (the total time will depend on the size and moisture content of the berries), stirring every 30 minutes or so, until the desired texture is reached. They should still be soft in the middle, but slightly shriveled and smaller than when you began. Allow to cool before using. Store, covered, in the refrigerator for up to 3 days, or freeze for later use.

Oven-Dried Tomatoes
Good for: all stages

These tomatoes are a great substitute for sun-dried tomatoes, which aren't permitted on the ACD. Because they take a while to bake, they're best made when you know you'll be home for a while; just pop them in the oven and go about your daily business while they dry.

MAKES ABOUT 2 CUPS (480 ML) TOMATOES

1 tablespoon (15 ml) extra-virgin olive oil or melted coconut
    oil, preferably organic
4 cups (1 L) grape tomatoes
Fine sea salt

Preheat the oven to 250°F (121°C). Line two large, rimmed cookie sheets with parchment.

In a large bowl, toss the tomatoes with the oil. Spread them evenly on the prepared cookie sheets, taking care that they are in a single layer and don't overlap. Sprinkle liberally with salt.

Bake for 2 to 3 hours, checking periodically, until the tomatoes are wrinkled and shrink down to about half their size. Allow to cool before using. Store, covered, in the refrigerator for up to 5 days, or freeze for later use.

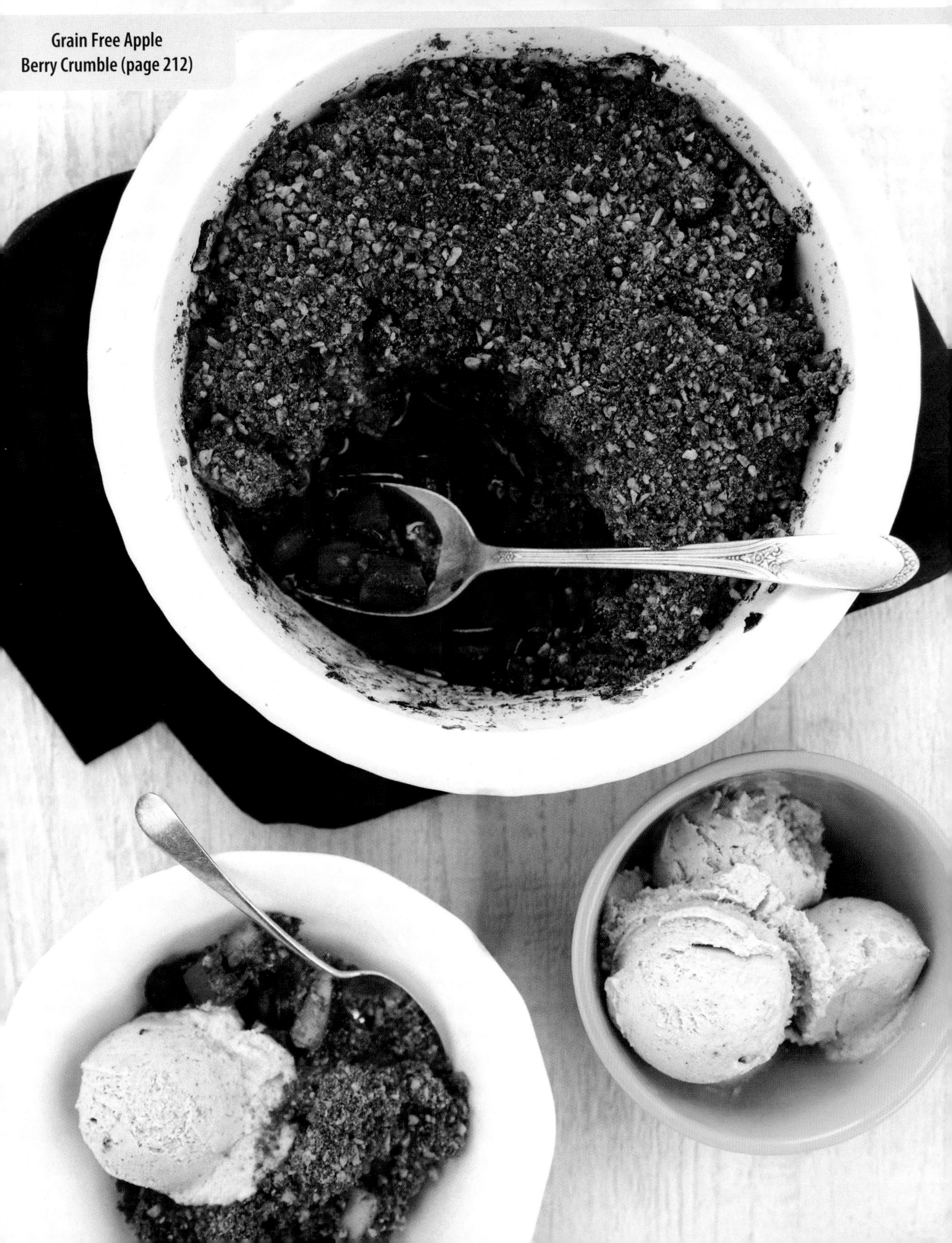
Grain Free Apple Berry Crumble (page 212)

"Sour Cream and Onion"
Kale Chips (page 139)

Sunday Night Roast (page 196) with
Perfect Golden Gravy (page 177)

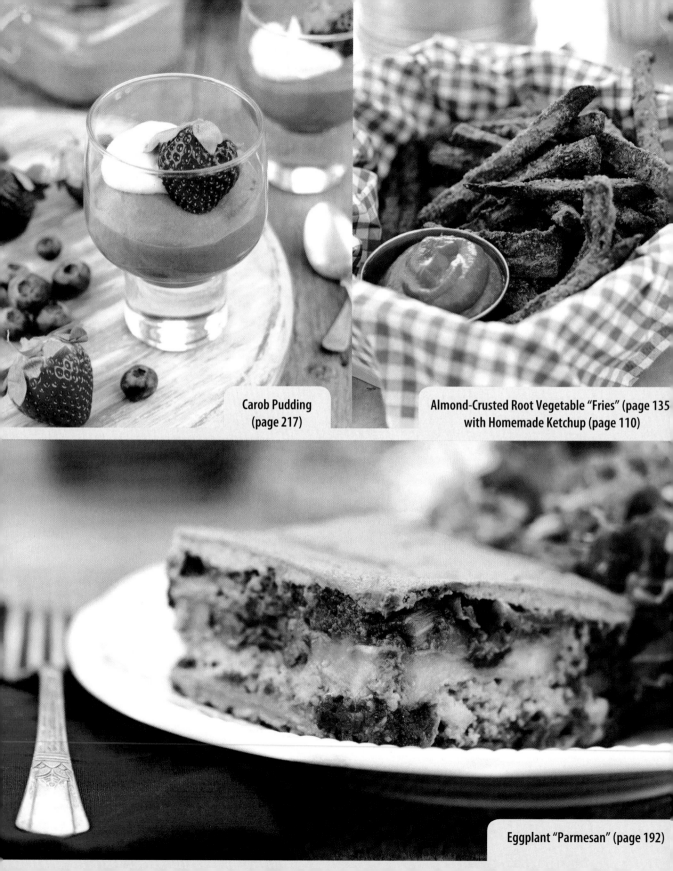

Carob Pudding
(page 217)

Almond-Crusted Root Vegetable "Fries" (page 135)
with Homemade Ketchup (page 110)

Eggplant "Parmesan" (page 192)

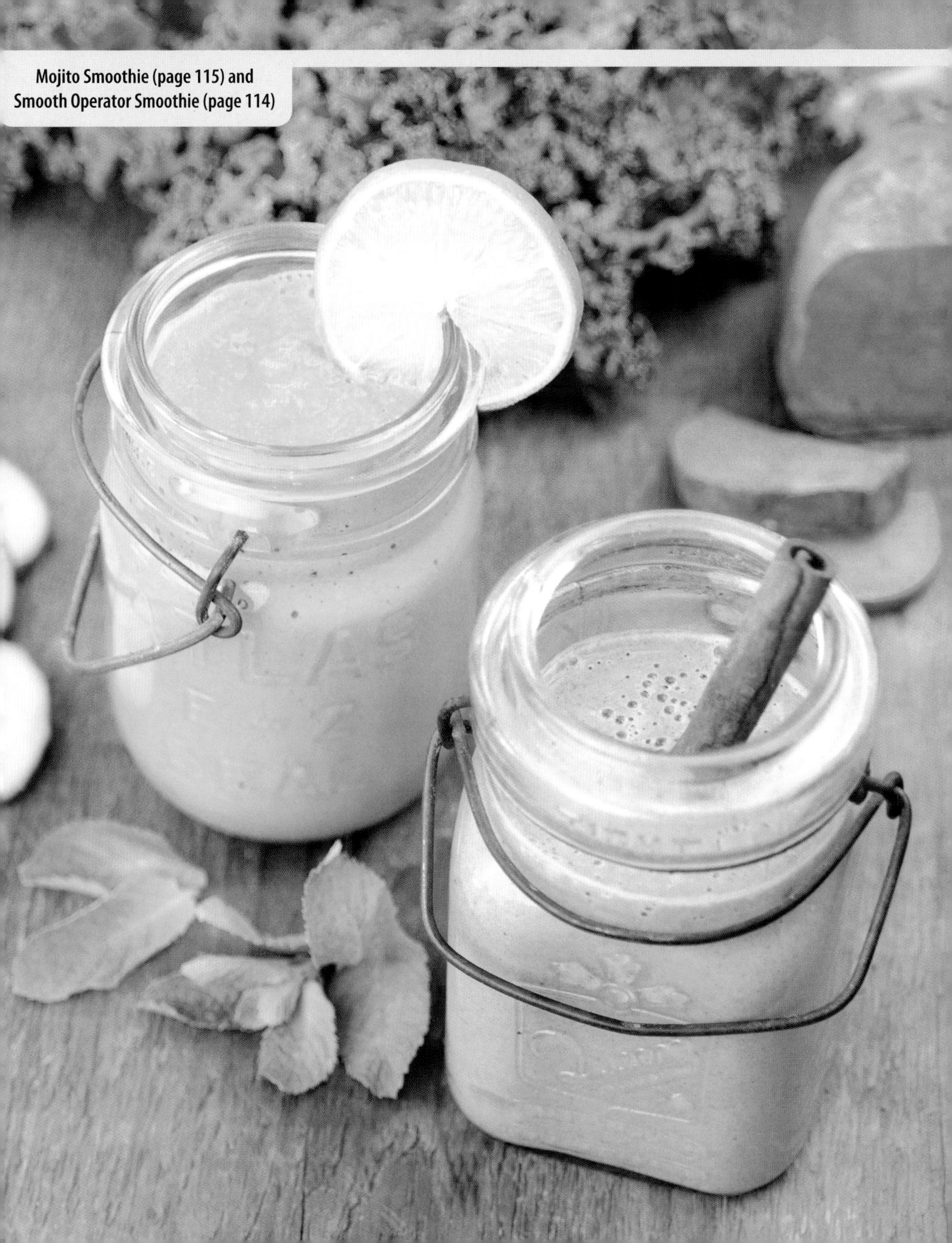

Mojito Smoothie (page 115) and
Smooth Operator Smoothie (page 114)

The "Toronto" Sandwich (page 151) with
As-You-Like Kale Salad (page 172) and
Garlicky Warm Avocado Sauce (page 179)

Raw Chocolate Chip Cookie
Dough Truffles (page 209)

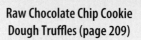

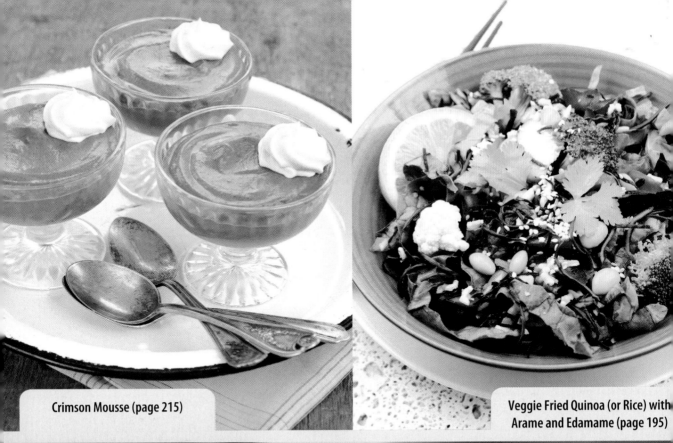

Crimson Mousse (page 215)

Veggie Fried Quinoa (or Rice) with Arame and Edamame (page 195)

Grain-Free Fudgy Brownies (page 206) with Vanilla Ice Cream (page 220)

ACD-Friendly Grain-Free
Granola (page 123)

Roasted Garlic and Cauliflower
Soup (page 147) with Grain-Free
Sandwich Bread (page 102)

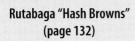
Rutabaga "Hash Browns"
(page 132)

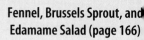

Fennel, Brussels Sprout, and Edamame Salad (page 166)

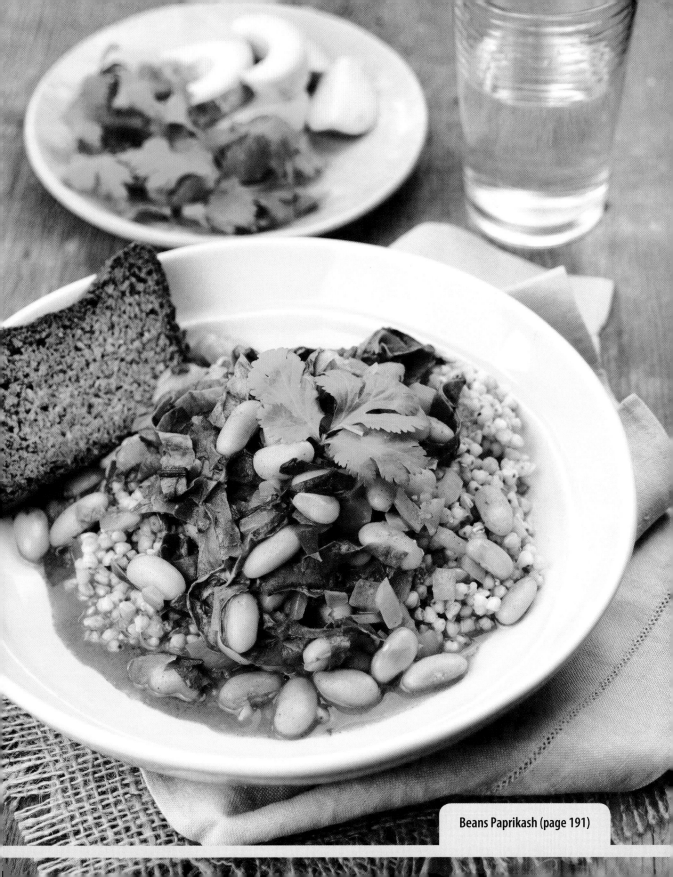

Beans Paprikash (page 191)

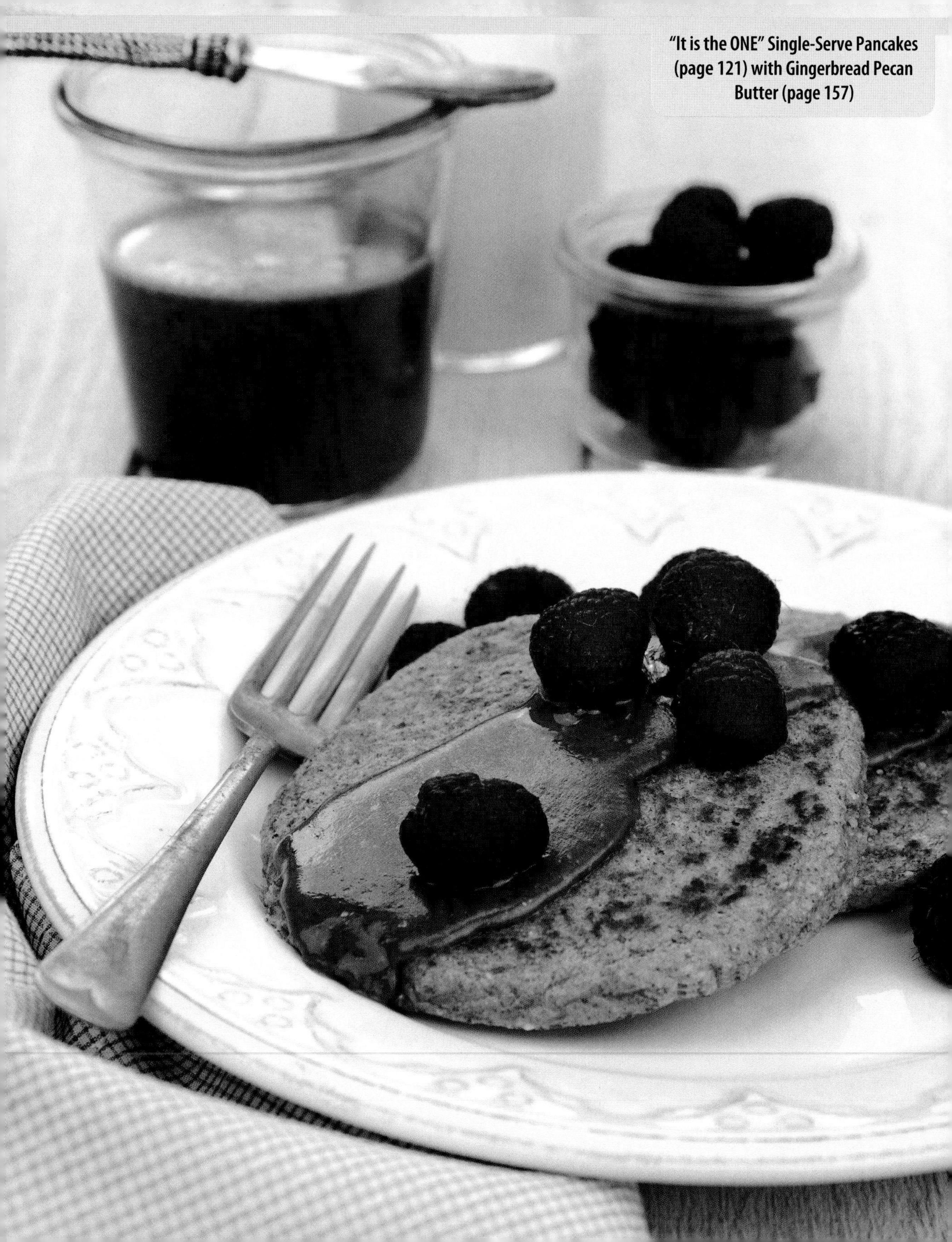
"It is the ONE" Single-Serve Pancakes (page 121) with Gingerbread Pecan Butter (page 157)

Quick and Easy Chard and
Chickpea Soup (page 149) with
Caesar Salad (page 175)

Tempeh "Bourguignon"
(page 198)

Raw Sushi with Spicy Ginger-
Miso Sauce (page 183)

Meaty Crumbles
Good for: all stages

This is one of my favorite recipes and a reader favorite on my blog as well. What starts out as lowly cauliflower is magically transformed in the oven to crumbles that eerily resemble ground beef in appearance, taste, and texture. These are incredibly versatile and can be used sprinkled on pizza crust, with sauce over pasta, as a filling for the "Toronto" Sandwich (page 151), in burritos, over nachos, shaped into patties and baked—basically, anywhere you'd use cooked ground beef.

MAKES ABOUT 6 CUPS (1.5 L) CRUMBLES

Nonstick spray (optional)
1 medium-size head cauliflower, trimmed and washed, broken
    into florets (about 1 pound [450 g] after trimming)
2 cups (250 g) raw walnut halves
2 tablespoons (30 ml) extra-virgin olive oil, preferably organic
2 garlic cloves, minced, or 1 teaspoon (5 ml) garlic powder
¼ teaspoon (1 ml) dried sage
1 teaspoon (5 ml) smoked paprika (see note)
½ to ¾ teaspoon (2.5 to 3.5 ml) fine sea salt
2 tablespoons (30 ml) Bragg Liquid Aminos (for soy-free, use
    coconut aminos)

Preheat the oven to 350°F (180°C). Line a large, rimmed cookie sheet or rectangular pan with parchment, or spray with nonstick spray.

Using a food processor, process the cauliflower and walnuts to a fine meal. Depending on how grainy you like your "meat," it can be more or less fine; I like mine similar to coarse cornmeal or finely chopped nuts.

Transfer the mixture to a large bowl and add the remaining ingredients.

Using clean hands, knead everything together thoroughly until the cauliflower mixture is uniformly coated.

Turn the mixture into the prepared pan and spread out evenly. Bake for 45 minutes and up to 1 hour 15 minutes (it will depend on the size of the pan and how thick the mixture is when you first begin to bake it), stirring after 30 minutes and then every 15 minutes after that, until the meat is dry and brown throughout. If you stir the crumbles and the layer underneath still looks wet and pale (as cauliflower tends to do), then bake for another 15 minutes before checking again. The crumbles will begin to separate and intensify in color as they roast.

Once the "meat" is cooked, you can cool, package, and freeze it for later use, or use it right away. It will keep, covered, in the refrigerator, for up to 3 days. May be frozen.

Basic Vegetable Broth or Stock
Good for: all stages

Many of my recipes call for vegetable broth or stock. I try to keep some home-made broth on hand at all times in the freezer, and this recipe is so easy to make, I often let it simmer while I'm cooking something else, then freeze in ice cube trays for later use (once frozen, pop out the cubes and store in a container in the freezer).

MAKES ABOUT 6 CUPS (1.5 L) BROTH

4 to 6 cups (1 to 1.5 L) mixed vegetable trimmings (from broccoli, carrot, celery, onion, stems from greens, rutabaga, cabbage, etc.—any odds and ends from vegetables that can be cooked)

1 whole onion, ends trimmed but with skin on (this adds a lovely color to the broth)

4 garlic cloves, peeled

1 bay leaf

1 carrot, peeled and cut into chunks

1 celery stalk, cut into chunks

1 small or ½ large tomato, cut into chunks

½ cup (120 ml) chopped fresh herbs (e.g., parsley, cilantro, oregano, basil, chives)

Place all the ingredients in a large pot with 10 cups (2.4 L) of filtered water and bring to a boil. Lower the heat and simmer until the vegetables are very soft and falling apart, for about 2 hours. If necessary, top up the water so that the pot is at least two-thirds full. Strain and reserve the broth. Discard or compost any solids.

Homemade Sauerkraut
Good for: all stages

When I first learned to make homemade sauerkraut in a raw foods class, I was amazed at how easy it was. Although there are many good-quality brands of lacto-fermented sauerkraut on the market, I like homemade because I can control the salt levels or add extra vegetables if I wish. Note that vegetables must be organic or they won't ferment properly; and be sure that your hands and all equipment are very clean before you start!

MAKES 6 TO 8 CUPS (1.5 TO 2 L) SAUERKRAUT

1 small organic green cabbage, or half each green and red
    cabbage
1 organic carrot or beet (optional)
About 1 teaspoon (5 ml) fine sea salt
Pure filtered water

Wash three or four pint-size (500 ml) glass jars with lids in a dishwasher or in very hot water; rinse and allow to dry.

Remove four of the outside leaves from the cabbage and set aside.

Grate the vegetables, using the medium-size holes on a food processor or box grater and place in a large bowl. Add the salt and toss to coat. Set aside about 3 cups (720 ml) of the vegetables.

Pack the remaining vegetable mixture into the jars, leaving about 2 inches (5 cm) of empty space at the top of each jar.

Combine the reserved 3 cups (720 ml) of vegetables with 1½ cups (360 ml) of filtered water and blend in the food processor to create a slurry. Pour the slurry over the vegetables in the jars to ensure that all the cabbage is submerged under liquid. Finally, take the whole cabbage leaves and roll them up tightly, then pack them on top of the vegetables in the jar as a stopper to keep the vegetables submerged. Screw on the lids, but not too tightly (some of the gases will escape while the cabbage ferments).

Set the jars in a warm, dry place for up to 1 week. After about 5 days, you can open the jars and sniff to see whether the mixture smells fermented (slightly sour, but not in a foul way). If there is a foul odor, this means the sauerkraut has gone bad and shouldn't be eaten. Once it reaches the desired state of fermentation, store in the refrigerator for up to 1 month.

Homemade Ketchup
Good for: all stages

Most store-bought ketchup is loaded with sugar and a variety of artificial ingredients and preservatives. While you should stay away from the processed versions, you don't have to give up ketchup completely! This homemade version is slightly lighter in color but every bit as flavorful as the ones you're used to.

MAKES ABOUT 2 CUPS (480 ML) KETCHUP

12 large beefsteak tomatoes, washed well and cored (no need
    to peel), or 1 (28-ounce [796 ml]) can stewed tomatoes
3 tablespoons (45 ml) raw apple cider vinegar
Juice of ½ lemon
1 teaspoon (5 ml) onion powder
2 teaspoons (10 ml) garlic powder or granulated garlic
2 teaspoons (10 ml) dry mustard
¼ teaspoon (1 ml) ground allspice, or ⅛ teaspoon (0.5 ml)
    ground cloves
1 teaspoon (5 ml) ground cinnamon
1 teaspoon (5 ml) sweet paprika

¼ to ½ teaspoon (1 to 2.5 ml) fine sea salt
⅛ teaspoon (0.5 ml) pure stevia powder

Puree the tomatoes in a food processor or blender. Place in a large pot with the other ingredients. Bring to a boil over medium heat, then lower the heat and continue to cook, stirring more frequently toward the end, until very thick and water no longer pools when you stir and scrape across the bottom of the pot (this could take up to 2 hours). Allow to cool; if desired, blend again for a smoother texture. Store a little in the fridge in a glass jar, but pour the remaining ketchup into ice cube trays and freeze, pop out and store in resealable plastic bags in the freezer; use one or two at a time as needed.

Glazed Tempeh
Good for: all stages

Q&E

Glazing the tempeh by panfrying until the marinade is absorbed is a fairly quick and easy way to transform this food into a flavorful and versatile high-protein addition to your meals. When sliced thinly and panfried until crispy, the tempeh can be used in place of bacon in the Caesar Salad (page 175).

MAKES 4 SERVINGS

3 tablespoons (45 ml) Bragg Liquid Aminos or wheat-free
   tamari
1½ teaspoons (7.5 ml) smoked paprika
10 drops plain pure liquid stevia
1 tablespoon (15 ml) raw apple cider vinegar
1 tablespoon (15 ml) extra-virgin olive oil, preferably organic
10 large grape or cherry tomatoes, or 1 large tomato, chopped
2 garlic cloves, minced
Pinch of fine sea salt
⅓ cup (80 ml) filtered water
1 (12- to 16-ounce [375 to 400 g]) package tempeh

Blend all the ingredients, except the tempeh, in a blender until liquefied.

Cut the tempeh into thin strips lengthwise, about ¼ inch (6 mm) thick (the number of strips will depend on your block of tempeh).

Place the tempeh in a nonstick skillet and pour the liquid over it. Turn each piece of tempeh over a few times to coat on both sides. Cook over medium-low heat, flipping the tempeh periodically, until all of the marinade is evaporated and the tempeh begins to brown considerably, for 15 to 25 minutes. May be frozen.

CHAPTER 7

Smoothies and Drinks

Classic Green Smoothie

Q&E

Good for: Stage 2 and beyond

Green smoothies are such a staple in my house that I almost forget they may not be part of everyone's regular breakfast rotation! While I normally add more fresh greens than any other ingredient, if green smoothies are new to you, start with just a couple of leaves of kale or a handful of spinach and work up from there. Use this recipe as a template to add your own mix of greens and/or (ACD-friendly) fruits and protein sources as you become more familiar with what you like. I've found that the recipe works equally well with spinach or chard for the greens, peaches or nectarines for the fruit, or other nuts or seeds instead of hemp seeds.

MAKES 2 BREAKFAST SERVINGS OR 4 SNACK SERVINGS

2 kale leaves, washed, stems removed, and chopped (if you
    don't have a powerful blender, use about 1 cup [240 ml]
    unpacked baby spinach instead)
1 cup (240 ml) fresh or frozen mixed berries (I use blueberries,
    blackberries, raspberries, and strawberries)
1 frozen pear, cored (you can leave the skin on)
¼ cup (40 g) raw shelled hemp seeds (hemp hearts)

¼ teaspoon (1 ml) plain or fruit-flavored pure liquid stevia, or
    to taste (about 40 drops)

2 tablespoons (30 ml) freshly squeezed lime juice (about ½
    lime)

2 tablespoons (30 ml) chia seeds (if using a regular blender,
    grind the seeds to a powder first in a coffee grinder)

1 to 2 teaspoons (5 to 10 ml) ground cinnamon

1 teaspoon (5 ml) pure vanilla extract (optional)

2 cups (480 ml) unsweetened almond, hemp, or Homemade
    Coconut Milk (page 99)

½ cup (120 ml) water, or more, to achieve desired consistency
    (use ice instead if your fruit isn't frozen)

Combine all the ingredients in a powerful blender and blend until smooth.

Smooth Operator Smoothie
Good for: all stages

Q&E

Smoothies are one of my favorite quick breakfasts that are also great to take along with you. This one, with sweet potato, greens, and seeds, provides all three macronutrients in one for a satisfying, nutritious start to your day.

MAKES 1 BREAKFAST SERVING OR 2 SNACK SERVINGS

1 cup (240 ml) kale, spinach, or romaine lettuce leaves

½ cup (120 ml) baked sweet potato or cooked squash, mashed
    or pureed

1 cup (240 ml) allowed alternative milk of choice

1 tablespoon (15 ml) ground flaxseeds, or 2 teaspoons (10 ml)
    ground chia seeds

2 teaspoons (10 ml) ground cinnamon

¼ teaspoon (1 ml) ground ginger, or 1 teaspoon (5 ml) grated
    fresh

15 to 25 drops plain or vanilla pure liquid stevia, or to taste

2 tablespoons (30 ml) raw shelled hemp seeds (hemp hearts)
   or pumpkin seeds

2 to 3 teaspoons (10 to 15 ml) freshly squeezed lime juice, to
   taste

½ cup (120 ml) ice (optional)

Blend all the ingredients until smooth. Enjoy.

Q&E

Mojito Smoothie
Good for: all stages

Traditional mojitos, of course, are off the table on an anticandida diet. This one provides the classic flavor combination in a beverage that will leave you refreshed and nourished instead of dehydrated or hung over. Sounds like a great trade to me! It's also a creamy, rich-tasting drink that will satisfy a sweet craving beautifully.

MAKES 1 LARGE OR 2 SMALLER SERVINGS

⅓ English cucumber, peeled and diced

4 curly kale leaves, stems removed

Juice and zest of ½ lime

10 to 15 drops plain or vanilla pure liquid stevia

½ large, barely ripe avocado (it should be quite firm), pitted
   and scooped from peel

15 to 20 mint leaves, or to taste; or ¼ to ½ teaspoon (1 to
   2.5 ml) pure peppermint extract

1 cup (240 ml) filtered water, or ½ cup (120 ml) water and ½
   cup (120 ml) full-fat canned coconut milk (for a creamier
   smoothie)

About ½ cup (120 ml) ice

In a strong blender, blend all the ingredients until smooth. Drink immediately.

Q&E   Protein-Boost Cranberry Smoothie
Good for: all stages

This is a quick and not-too-filling smoothie that's great for an afternoon snack.

MAKES 1 SERVING

¾ to 1 cup (180 to 240 ml) unsweetened almond, hemp, or
    other milk of choice
2 tablespoons (30 ml) unflavored or vanilla protein powder (for
    Stage 1, use hemp protein; otherwise, pea or rice is fine)
1 teaspoon (5 ml) lemon or lime zest
6 tablespoons (90 ml) Coconut-Cranberry Spread (page 158)
Stevia (optional)
1 teaspoon (5 ml) pure vanilla extract (optional)

Place all the ingredients in a blender and blend until smooth. Enjoy.

Q&E   ACD-Friendly Fruity Sipper—hot or cold
Good for: all stages

This recipe was inspired by a cider drink on my friend Lexie's blog (*Lexie's Kitchen*). My cold version is reminiscent of that familiar childhood drink filled with artificial colors, flavors, and loads of sugar—but this one is actually good for you! It tastes tart, sweet, and fruity all at the same time. In colder months, I enjoy a steaming cup of Fruity Sipper almost every evening; it's a perfect way to wind down after a long day.

MAKES 1 SERVING

1 fruit-flavored herbal tea bag of choice (I love ginger-peach,
    lemon ginger, blueberry, mixed fruit, or apple-cinnamon)
1¾ cups (420 ml) boiling water
2 teaspoons (10 ml) raw apple cider vinegar
Stevia

In a large mug, steep the tea bag in the boiling water for 5 minutes. Remove the tea bag and add the vinegar and stevia to taste. Sip and enjoy!

Note: For a cold drink, steep the tea bag in ½ cup (120 ml) of boiling water for 10 minutes. Remove the tea bag, then add ¾ cup (90 ml) of cold water and ½ cup (120 ml) of ice along with the vinegar and stevia.

Q&E

Sparkling Cranberry Cooler
Good for: all stages

I love this drink in the summer, or any time I want a beverage that feels festive and celebratory. While your friends sip on alcoholic drinks, this is a great option that allows you to remain on the diet. It looks lovely in a champagne flute, too.

MAKES 1 LARGE SERVING

¼ cup (60 ml) unsweetened cranberry juice
Juice of ½ lime
1¾ to 2 cups (420 to 480 ml) sparkling mineral water (not club
    soda)
Stevia
Ice (optional)

Combine all the ingredients in a tall glass, including stevia to taste, and stir gently to mix. Add ice, if desired, and sip happily.

CHAPTER 8

Breakfast

ACD Whole-Grain Waffles
Good for: all stages

Q&E

I find waffles are perfect for brunch, when you have a little more time in the morning to use a waffle iron. These are made with whole grains and added protein from the chickpea flour. I usually cook a double batch, then freeze leftovers for another day. These are lovely served with High-Protein Carob-Hazelnut Butter (page 155), Coconut-Cranberry Spread (page 158), or any nut butter of choice. For savory sandwiches, leave out the stevia and use your waffles instead of bread.

MAKES 4 TO 5 LARGE ROUND WAFFLES

½ cup (90 g) raw or toasted buckwheat groats
⅔ cup (130 g) uncooked millet
2 tablespoons (30 ml) psyllium husks
2 tablespoons (30 ml) chickpea flour
1 tablespoon (15 ml) ground flaxseeds (about 1½ teaspoons
    [7.5 ml] whole seeds)
1 teaspoon (5 ml) baking powder
⅛ teaspoon (0.5 ml) fine sea salt
1¾ cups (420 ml) unsweetened nondairy milk of choice, plus
    up to ¼ cup (60 ml) more, if needed

10 drops plain or vanilla pure liquid stevia
1 teaspoon (5 ml) raw apple cider vinegar
2 tablespoons (30 ml) coconut oil, preferably organic

Place all the ingredients in a high-powered blender and blend until combined. The batter will be very thick, like a muffin batter; if it is really too thick, add a bit more milk. Allow to sit for 2 minutes. Grease and heat the waffle iron according to the manufacturer's directions. Using a large ice-cream scoop, scoop batter onto the iron and allow to cook until quite browned. You can keep the waffles warm on a parchment-lined cookie sheet or heatproof plate at 275°F (135°C) while you continue with the rest of the batter. May be frozen.

Note: This batter does not work for pancakes. If you prefer pancakes for breakfast, see the Fluffy Pancakes recipe (page 120) instead.

Fluffy Pancakes
Good for: all stages

Q&E

Pancakes are, hands-down, my favorite breakfast food. In fact, they're probably one of my favorite lunch and dinner foods, too! These are a classic version; the millet and coconut flour create a dry, light interior and cakey texture. I love them with some melted Gingerbread Pecan Butter (page 157) or Classic Whipped Cream (page 221) on top.

MAKES 4 PANCAKES

¼ cup (60 ml) uncooked millet
2 tablespoons (30 ml) Garfava or chickpea flour
2 tablespoons (30 ml) coconut flour
2 teaspoons (10 ml) whole psyllium husks
1 tablespoon (15 ml) finely ground flaxseeds
½ teaspoon (2.5 ml) baking powder
¼ teaspoon (1 ml) baking soda
Pinch of fine sea salt

¾ cup (180 ml) unsweetened almond milk or Homemade
   Coconut Milk (page 99)
2 teaspoons (10 ml) raw apple cider vinegar
1 teaspoon (5 ml) pure vanilla extract
10 to 15 drops plain or vanilla pure liquid stevia, or more to
   taste
Nonstick spray or coconut oil, for pan (optional)
Nut butter or other topping, for serving

In a coffee grinder or blender, blend the millet and Garfava flour to a fine powder. Place in a bowl with the coconut flour, psyllium, flax, baking powder, baking soda, and salt; stir to combine.

Add the milk, vinegar, vanilla, and stevia, and stir until blended; do not overmix. Allow to sit for 2 minutes undisturbed.

Heat a nonstick skillet over medium heat (if necessary, spray or grease the pan). Use a large ice-cream scoop or ⅓ cup (80 ml) measuring cup to scoop the batter and place it in the pan. It will be thick and you may need to gently spread it out with a spatula to form the pancakes.

Cook for 4 to 5 minutes, until the tops are almost completely dry and the bottoms are deep golden brown, then gently flip and continue to cook for another 3 to 4 minutes until browned on the other side. Top with your desired topping. May be frozen.

Q&E "It Is the ONE" Single-Serve Pancakes
Good for: all stages

Looking for a filling, hot breakfast on a workday morning? These single-serve pancakes are ready in less than ten minutes. And the recipe is so easy to remember—1 tablespoon (15 ml) of just about every ingredient!

MAKES 1 SERVING

6 tablespoons (75 ml) allowed milk of choice (unsweetened
   almond, hemp, flax, etc.)
1 teaspoon (5 ml) raw apple cider vinegar
5 to 10 drops plain or vanilla pure liquid stevia, or to taste
1 tablespoon (15 ml) smooth natural almond butter or
   sunflower seed butter
1 tablespoon (15 ml) whole chia seeds
1 tablespoon (15 ml) uncooked quinoa, millet, or amaranth
1 tablespoon (15 ml) uncooked whole buckwheat
1 tablespoon (15 ml) raw shelled hemp seeds (hemp hearts)
1 tablespoon (15 ml) coconut flour
¼ teaspoon (1 ml) baking powder
Pinch of fine sea salt
Coconut oil, for pan (optional)

In a medium-size bowl, whisk together the milk, vinegar, stevia, and almond butter until smooth. Set aside.

In a coffee grinder or blender, grind the chia, quinoa, buckwheat, hemp seeds, coconut flour, baking powder, and salt to a powder. Pour the mixture over the wet ingredients in the bowl and stir to blend. It will seem a bit too thick for pancake batter and more like a soft cookie dough. This is as it should be.

Heat a nonstick skillet over medium heat (brush with coconut oil if it has a tendency to stick). Divide the batter in half and place in the skillet (I use an ice-cream scoop), then use a spatula to flatten to about ¼ inch (6 mm) thick. Cook until the top begins to dry out (about 4 minutes); flip and cook for another 3 to 4 minutes. Serve immediately. May be prepared in advance and frozen. Will keep, frozen, for up to 3 months.

ACD-Friendly Grain-Free Granola
Good for: all stages

If you're a fan of cold cereals, you don't have to miss out when following the early stages of the diet. This granola fits the bill perfectly: it bakes up in little clusters that are browned and crispy, and they stay that way in milk. The recipe requires a bit of time to prepare, but, once it's done, you'll have a large batch of granola that will stay fresh for up to a week in a covered container.

MAKES 6 SERVINGS

1 medium-size zucchini, peeled and cut into chunks (7¾ ounces [220 g] as chunks; see note)

2 tablespoons (30 ml) smooth natural almond butter or sunflower seed butter

2 tablespoons (30 ml) water

2 tablespoons (30 ml) yacon syrup

½ teaspoon (2.5 ml) plain or vanilla pure liquid stevia (about 40 drops), or more to taste

6 tablespoons (60 g) finely ground chia seeds (from about 3 tablespoons [45 ml] whole seeds)

5 ounces (145 g) unsweetened medium-shred coconut (about 1½ cups)

1½ tablespoons (22.5 ml) ground cinnamon

½ teaspoon (2.5 ml) ground ginger, or 2 teaspoons (10 ml) grated fresh

1 teaspoon (5 ml) pure vanilla powder, or 2 teaspoons (10 ml) pure vanilla extract

2 tablespoons (30 ml) lightly toasted or raw sesame seeds

2 tablespoons (30 ml) sunflower seeds

2 tablespoons (30 ml) pumpkin seeds

Additions for later stages: goji berries, golden berries, or chopped prunes (see note)

¼ cup (60 ml) lightly toasted or raw walnut or pecan pieces

¼ cup (60 ml) coarsely chopped, lightly toasted or raw hazelnuts or almonds

Preheat the oven to 350°F (180°C). Line a large pan (e.g., a lasagna pan) with parchment.

In the bowl of a food processor, blend the zucchini, almond butter, water, yacon, and stevia until liquefied. Add the chia, coconut, cinnamon, ginger, and vanilla and blend again until the mixture resembles a sticky dough. Allow to sit for 5 minutes to thicken up.

Using your hands, crumble the dough into clumps and spread evenly over the prepared cookie sheet. Bake for 30 minutes, then remove from the oven and stir gently with a spatula, flipping over as many pieces as you can (they should be starting to dry out and no longer stick together).

Decrease the oven temperature to 325°F (170°C). Bake the granola for another 30 to 40 minutes, stirring every 15 minutes or so, until the mixture is dry and dark brown in places. Turn off the heat and leave the granola in the oven to cool (prop the door open slightly while cooling).

Once cool, check to ensure that the granola is dried through and crispy. If not, bake for another 20 minutes at 325°F (170°C) and cool again.

To the crisp granola, add the seeds, fruit, if using, and nuts. Stir to combine. Store in an airtight container for up to 1 week. Serve with your milk of choice, or eat as a snack. Cooled granola can be stored in a sealed container at room temperature for up to 1 week, or in the refrigerator for up to 2 weeks.

Note: In later stages of the diet, once you add fruit back to your diet, you can substitute ½ cup (120 ml) of unsweetened applesauce for the zucchini, or add goji berries, golden berries, or dried prunes to your bowl.

Raw Apple Porridge Bowl
Good for: Stage 2 and beyond

Q&E

I try to eat raw foods at least 50 percent of the time, either as half my plate or for half my meals. This number increases in the summer with the abundance of fresh produce everywhere. This raw porridge provides a nice light breakfast that's surprisingly satisfying, and it's perfect for those months when you don't want to heat up the kitchen.

MAKES 1 LARGE SERVING

1 medium-size apple, quartered and cored
½ small beet, peeled, finely grated (optional)
1 tablespoon (15 ml) chia seeds, ground to a powder in a
    coffee grinder
1 tablespoon (15 ml) ground flaxseeds
1 tablespoon (15 ml) sunflower or pumpkin seeds
1 tablespoon (15 ml) unsweetened shredded coconut
1 teaspoon (5 ml) grated fresh ginger
1 teaspoon (5 ml) ground cinnamon
About ½ cup (120 ml) unsweetened almond, hemp, flax, or
    other allowed milk of choice, plus more, if desired
5 to 10 drops plain or vanilla pure liquid stevia, or to taste

Either dice or grate the apple and place half in a bowl with the grated beet, if using. Place the other half of the apple in a small food processor with the remaining ingredients and blend until almost smooth. Once combined, add to the bowl along with extra milk, if desired. Eat immediately (this does not keep well).

Baked Quinoa Porridge or Pudding
Good for: all stages

I love baked oatmeal, so was delighted to find a way to reproduce the creaminess of oatmeal in a quinoa-based porridge. Top with a dollop of Vanilla Ice Cream (page 220) or Classic Whipped Cream (page 221) and the recipe serves as a lovely, not-too-sweet dessert as well. It also tastes great cold from the refrigerator the next day.

MAKES 4 TO 6 SERVINGS

Coconut oil, for pan
½ cup (95 g) uncooked quinoa (either soak overnight or rinse if
     dry; see soaking guidelines, page 95).
⅓ cup (80 ml) smooth natural almond butter (or use another
     nut butter if you prefer)
1½ cups (360 ml) unsweetened plain or vanilla almond, or
     hemp milk, or Homemade Coconut Milk (page 99)
2 teaspoons (10 ml) pure vanilla extract
1 tablespoon (15 ml) ground cinnamon
2 teaspoons (10 ml) minced fresh ginger, or ¾ teaspoon
     (3.5 ml) ground
Pinch of fine sea salt
1/16 teaspoon (0.25 ml) pure stevia powder, or ⅛ teaspoon
     (0.5 ml) pure liquid stevia, or to taste

Preheat the oven to 350°F (180°C). Grease a medium-size (about 6 cups [1.5 L]) lidded casserole dish.

Sprinkle the quinoa into the prepared dish. In a medium-size bowl, whisk together the remaining ingredients until smooth, then pour over the quinoa. Stir gently until all the quinoa is submerged under the liquid. Cover and bake for 30 minutes.

Remove from the oven, uncover, and stir; replace the cover, and continue to bake, checking every 20 minutes or so, until the liquid is absorbed and the porridge is cooked and creamy, for 40 to 50 more minutes. Spoon into bowls and serve (this is lovely with ice cream or whipped cream).

Variations: After mixing everything in the casserole dish, add up to ½ cup (120 ml) total of any one of the following (or a combination totaling ½ cup [120 ml]): walnuts, pecans, pumpkin seeds, sunflower seeds, or Oven-Dried Cranberries (page 105) at any stage; or blueberries, raspberries, blackberries, or chopped apple or pear at Stage 2 or beyond.

Almost Instant Grain-Free Breakfast Porridge
Good for: Stage 2 and beyond (or all stages if fruit is omitted)

Q&E

I came across this recipe when I first taught a course with Andrea and it was included in the recipe packet for course participants. It was definitely love at first bite! This porridge is quick and easy, and infinitely variable: use sunflower or hemp instead of the pumpkin seeds; substitute another favorite nut instead of the walnuts; include the coconut or omit it, as you wish. It's also a great year-round breakfast as you won't have to heat up the kitchen cooking it on the stove top.

MAKES 1 SERVING

2 tablespoons (30 ml) unsweetened coconut flakes or shredded
    coconut
1 tablespoon (15 ml) raw pumpkin seeds
1 tablespoon (15 ml) raw whole flaxseeds
2 teaspoons (10 ml) chia seeds
1 tablespoon (15 ml) raw walnuts (about 6 walnuts)
½ teaspoon (2.5 ml) ground cinnamon
½ to ¾ cup (120 to 180 ml) very hot water
7 to 10 drops plain or vanilla pure liquid stevia
2 to 4 tablespoons (30 to 60 ml) Homemade Coconut Milk
    (page 99), almond, or other milk of choice
½ cup (120 ml) blueberries or other fresh berries, or chopped
    fresh apricots

In a coffee grinder, grind the coconut, pumpkin seeds, flaxseeds, chia seeds, walnuts, and cinnamon. Transfer to a bowl and cover with water. Let sit for a few minutes to thicken.

Add the stevia, coconut milk, and blueberries and stir well.

Note: You can make a large batch of this cereal in advance and store it in single servings in the freezer so it's ready to go when you need it: thaw overnight in the refrigerator and enjoy! It's also great for traveling. Just bring single servings of the dry mixture with you in resealable plastic bags, empty into a bowl, and add hot water for a quick and delicious breakfast.

Chia-Rice Pudding (or Breakfast)
Good for: all stages

Q&E

Chia is packed with healthy omega-3 fats and protein, a perfect balance to the complex carbohydrates in the rice. This is a supernutritious breakfast, but one sweet enough to double as dessert!

MAKES 4 TO 6 SERVINGS

1 cup (240 ml) canned organic full-fat coconut milk, or more if desired
1 cup (240 ml) filtered water or unsweetened almond milk
2 cups (480 ml) cold cooked brown rice (a great use for leftover rice!)
2 teaspoons (10 ml) pure vanilla extract, or 1 teaspoon (5 ml) vanilla powder
⅛ teaspoon (0.5 ml) pure stevia powder, or ¼ teaspoon (1 ml) pure liquid stevia (I like toffee flavor), or to taste
2 teaspoons (10 ml) ground cinnamon
Pinch of fine sea salt
⅓ cup (55 g) whole chia seeds
Additional ground cinnamon, for sprinkling

In a medium-size pot, bring the coconut milk, water, rice, vanilla, stevia, cinnamon, and salt to a boil. Remove from the heat immediately and allow to cool, uncovered, for about 5 minutes.

Pour into a heatproof bowl. Add the chia and stir to combine. Allow to cool to room temperature, stirring one or two times to break up any clumps formed by the chia. Once cool, store in a covered container in the refrigerator. To serve, stir again (adding more milk if necessary to achieve desired texture), scoop into serving bowls, and sprinkle with cinnamon. Leftovers will keep, covered in the refrigerator, for up to 4 days.

Sweet Potato Rounds with Sweet or Savory Almond Sauce
Good for: all stages

You may not necessarily think of sweet potato as a breakfast food, but this hearty, easy recipe satisfies the taste buds and the belly! When I first started an anticandida diet, baked sweet potato with sweet almond sauce was one of my favorite breakfasts. This supereasy recipe is a great side dish, too.

MAKES 1 SERVING

1 sweet potato (peel if desired)
1 recipe Sweet or Savory Almond Sauce (page 178)

Preheat the oven to 400°F (200°C). Place the whole sweet potato on a parchment-lined cookie sheet and bake until very soft for about 1 hour. Remove from the oven and slice into large rounds about 1 inch (2.5 cm) thick to serve, or, for an easier preparation, simply slice the sweet potato in half lengthwise. Top with your sauce of choice and enjoy! Note: The sweet potato is equally tasty at room temperature (so you can bake it in advance and eat it later). Will keep, covered, in the refrigerator for up to 2 days.

Zucchini Fritters
Q&E
Good for: all stages

A quick and easy savory alternative to weekend pancakes. While these fritters have the same light, airy base as a traditional cake, the zucchini lends moistness and a mildly savory overtone. Paired with some nut butter and a green salad, these are also perfect for a light lunch.

MAKES 5 TO 6 FRITTERS

1 large zucchini, unpeeled
About 2 teaspoons (10 ml) fine sea salt
½ cup (50 g) chickpea flour
½ teaspoon (2.5 ml) dried tarragon
4 teaspoons (20 ml) black or white sesame seeds
¼ teaspoon (1 ml) baking powder
⅛ teaspoon (0.5 ml) baking soda
⅓ cup (80 ml) drained zucchini juice (see directions) plus water
    and/or vegetable broth, as needed
2 teaspoons (10 ml) freshly squeezed lemon juice

Wash and trim the zucchini and grate medium-fine. Set a colander or sieve above a large bowl and place the zucchini in the colander. Sprinkle with salt and toss lightly. Allow the zucchini to rest for at least 10 minutes so that the salt will extract the excess moisture from the zucchini. Then squeeze the zucchini to remove as much liquid as you can (allow the juice to drain into the bowl). Reserve the zucchini juice.

While the zucchini rests, place the flour, tarragon, sesame seeds, baking powder, and baking soda in a medium-size bowl and whisk to combine. Pour the reserved zucchini liquid into a glass measuring cup and add water as necessary to make ⅓ cup (80 ml). Add the lemon juice to the cup.

Turn the drained zucchini into the bowl with the flour and add the liquids. Stir quickly to combine, but don't overstir.

Heat a nonstick skillet over medium heat. Using a large ice-cream scoop or ⅓ cup (80 ml) measuring cup, scoop the batter into the pan, and flatten slightly to create pancakes. Allow to cook for 4 to 5 minutes, until the tops are almost dry and the bottoms are browned. Flip and cook for another 3 to 4 minutes. Will keep, covered in the refrigerator, for up to 4 days. May be frozen.

Veggie-Full Breakfast Hash
Good for: all stages

A flavorful hash is practically a meal in itself. This recipe is perfect as the main dish for a weekend breakfast or brunch. The tempeh provides a great source of protein, and, paired with the sweet potato and other vegetables, there's also a great variety of colors, flavors, and textures, too.

MAKES 4 TO 6 SERVINGS

1 tablespoon (15 ml) extra-virgin olive oil, preferably organic

1 large onion, diced

2 celery stalks, diced

2 large carrots, grated

1 small green or red bell pepper, cored and diced

1 small jalapeño pepper, minced (remove seeds for less heat)

3 garlic cloves, minced

2 medium-size sweet potatoes (about 10.5 ounces [300 g]), peeled and diced into ½ inch (1.3 cm) cubes and boiled until barely tender, for about 5 minutes, then drained (see note)

¼ cup (60 ml) vegetable broth or water

1 teaspoon (5 ml) smoked paprika or ground cumin

1 teaspoon (5 ml) dried basil, or 1 tablespoon (15 ml) fresh

1 teaspoon (5 ml) dried dill, or 1 tablespoon (15 ml) fresh

3 to 4 tablespoons (45 to 60 ml) Bragg Liquid Aminos or wheat-free tamari, or to taste

Fine sea salt and freshly ground black pepper

½ cup (120 ml) chopped fresh parsley

1 block (1 pound or 400 to 500 g) tempeh, cut into small squares, or 2 cups (480 ml) cooked black beans, or a combination (marinated, leftover tempeh is fine in this)

1 avocado, peeled, pitted, and sliced, for topping (optional)

Heat the oil in a large skillet over medium heat. Add the onion, celery, carrot, and bell pepper and sauté until the onion is soft and translucent, for 5 to 7 minutes. Add the jalapeño and garlic and continue to cook for another 2 minutes, stirring often.

Add the remaining ingredients and stir gently to coat the tempeh and potatoes. Cover and cook until the onion is golden and the hash begins to brown on the bottom, for 10 to 20 minutes, stirring occasionally to prevent burning (timing will depend on your stove and the pan). Serve as is or at room temperature, topped with avocado slices, if desired. Will keep, covered in the refrigerator, for up to 4 days. May be frozen.

Note: If you're following the Fast Track version of the diet, you can omit the tempeh and replace the sweet potato with rutabaga; add nuts or seeds of choice to increase the protein content in this recipe.

Rutabaga "Hash Browns"
Good for: all stages

For those of you missing potatoes, these hash browns will fulfill those desires! Although this dish takes some time to cook fully, it's a really easy recipe to make, as you can more or less forget about it while it cooks, stirring only occasionally while you putter around in other parts of the house. As the vegetables begin to brown and caramelize, you'll find that the tantalizing aroma draws you back to the kitchen.

For early stages, omit the parsnip and use a bit more rutabaga.

MAKES 6 TO 8 SERVINGS

1 small rutabaga, peeled
1 small zucchini, trimmed (you can leave the skin on)
1 medium-size parsnip, peeled
1 large onion

½ cup (120 ml) chopped fresh herbs (I use a mixture of parsley
    and dill; cilantro is also nice)
6 garlic cloves, chopped
2 tablespoons (30 ml) extra-virgin olive oil, preferably organic
½ cup (120 ml) vegetable broth or stock
Fine sea salt (optional)

Grate the rutabaga, zucchini, parsnip, and onion, using the medium grater blade of a food processor. Otherwise, grate all the vegetables on the medium holes of a box grater.

Place the grated vegetables, herbs, garlic, and oil in a large, nonstick skillet at least 10 inches (25 cm) in diameter (a cast-iron pan is great for this recipe). Pour the broth evenly over the top and stir to mix. Place over medium-high heat and allow to cook until the mixture begins to sizzle and cook on the edges, for 15 to 25 minutes. Stir the vegetables to distribute any browned bits evenly throughout.

Cover the pan and lower the heat to medium-low. Allow to cook undisturbed for another 15 to 25 minutes, then check to see whether the veggies have begun to form a brown crust on the bottom. If they have, stir once more, taste and add salt, if desired, and then cook again for another 10 to 15 minutes, until cooked throughout and crusty in spots. Serve immediately. May be frozen.

Chickpea Breakfast Scramble
Good for: all stages

Q&E

Most vegan scrambles are made from tofu, an ingredient that some people prefer to avoid. I was delighted to discover that I could create an equally delicious as well as high-protein version by using chickpea flour. This scramble has become my quick, go-to scramble when I want something hearty in a jiffy on a weekday morning. For a complete meal, serve with a side salad and a slice of Grain-Free Sandwich Bread (page 102).

MAKES 2 SERVINGS

½ cup (50 g) chickpea flour
½ cup (120 ml) vegetable broth or stock
⅛ teaspoon (0.5 ml) ground turmeric (optional)
Pinch of fine sea salt, or to taste
½ medium-size tomato, chopped
½ small zucchini, diced
½ cup (120 ml) broccoli florets
1 teaspoon (5 ml) dried dill, 1 teaspoon (5 ml) dried parsley, or
    1 tablespoon (15 ml) chopped fresh parsley or cilantro, (see
    note)
1 tablespoon (15 ml) extra-virgin olive oil, preferably organic
½ medium-size onion, chopped

In a medium-size bowl, whisk together the chickpea flour, broth, turmeric, and salt until smooth. Add the tomato, zucchini, broccoli, and herb of choice and stir until the veggies are coated.

In a large, nonstick skillet, heat the oil over medium heat. Add the onion and sauté until translucent, for about 7 minutes. Add the chickpea mixture and stir once or twice, as you would scrambled eggs. Keep stirring as the mixture comes together, cutting large pieces with a wooden spoon or spatula to create a mixture that looks like scrambled eggs, for 5 to 8 minutes. Keep cooking until the "egg" mixture is dried throughout, for another 5 to 10 minutes.

Note: In general, use fresh herbs when you can get them; if all you have is dried, you can usually substitute 1 teaspoon (5 ml) dried per 1 tablespoon (15 ml) fresh for leafy herbs, such as parsley or cilantro.

CHAPTER 9

Sides and Snacks

Almond-Crusted Root Vegetable "Fries"
Good for: all stages

This recipe couldn't be simpler—and because it works with most root veggies, it's versatile, too. The only caveat is to be sure to bake the fries long enough, so that the coating becomes somewhat crispy; this isn't the time for mushy, just-done fries. When properly baked, the almond coating crisps up nicely, the fries themselves begin to caramelize and sweeten, and the whole package is entirely irresistible. These are great with Homemade Ketchup (page 110).

MAKES 3 TO 4 SERVINGS

Coconut oil, for pan (optional)
1 medium-size rutabaga, 3 medium-size parsnips, or 2
    medium-size sweet potatoes, or other root vegetables of
    your choice, peeled and cut into thin, frylike strips (or use a
    combination of those listed)
3 tablespoons (45 ml) smooth natural almond butter
1 tablespoon (15 ml) extra-virgin olive oil, preferably organic
½ teaspoon (2.5 ml) fine sea salt
About 1 teaspoon (5 ml) total spice(s) of your choice (garlic
    salt, curry powder, cumin, garam masala, Chinese 5-spice
    powder, etc.)

Preheat the oven to 400°F (200°C). Line a large baking sheet with parchment, or grease with coconut oil.

Place the "fries" in a large bowl. In a small bowl, combine the almond butter, oil, salt, and spices. Drizzle the coating over the fries, and toss the mixture with a large spoon (or even better, your hands) until they are all evenly coated.

Line up the fries on the baking sheet in a single layer. Bake for 50 to 70 minutes (depending on thickness of your fries), until the coating is browned and a bit crispy, and the fries are fully cooked. Will keep, refrigerated, for up to 3 days.

Roasted Roots
Good for: all stages

Jerusalem artichokes (also called sunchokes) are particularly beneficial on an anticandida diet, as they are a good source of inulin, a "prebiotic" that helps nourish the good bacteria in the gut. With a texture much like that of other root vegetables when baked, they also happen to taste great! If you can't find Jerusalem artichokes, you can leave them out and use extra celery root and/or rutabaga in this lovely side dish.

MAKES 3 TO 4 SERVINGS

1 large onion, cut into eighths
1 pound (500 g) Jerusalem artichokes, scrubbed and peeled (or unmarinated regular artichoke hearts, if desired)
1 medium-size celery root, trimmed and cut into 1-inch (2.5 cm) chunks
1 large red-skinned potato, scrubbed and cut into 1.5-inch (4 cm) chunks
½ medium-size rutabaga, peeled and diced into 1-inch (2.5 cm) chunks
2 tablespoons (30 ml) extra-virgin olive oil
1 to 2 tablespoons (15 to 30 ml) fresh or dried rosemary
Fine sea salt

Preheat the oven to 400°F (200°C). Place the veggies in a large casserole or rectangular baking pan and drizzle with the oil; toss to coat. Sprinkle with rosemary and salt.

Bake, uncovered, stirring two or three times during baking, until soft and browned, 40 minutes to an hour. Serve.

Cauliflower and Bean Mash
Good for: all stages

This is a great substitute for mashed potatoes, offering less starch and more protein than regular spuds. Serve this mash alongside Sunday Night Roast (page 196) or other entrée for a comforting and delicious side dish.

MAKES 4 TO 6 SERVINGS

½ large head cauliflower, washed, trimmed, and cut into
    florets (about 3 cups [720 ml])
2 tablespoons (30 ml) extra-virgin olive oil, plus up to 1
    tablespoon (15 ml) more, if needed
2 large garlic cloves, still in papery skins
¾ cup (180 ml) cooked great northern or navy beans
2 tablespoons (30 ml) tahini (sesame paste)
Fine sea salt and freshly ground black pepper

Preheat the oven to 400°F (200°C). In a large rectangular pan (a lasagna pan works nicely for this), toss the cauliflower with the olive oil. Spread the mixture evenly in the pan, keeping it in a single layer as much as possible. Place the garlic cloves in the pan.

Bake, uncovered, for 30 to 40 minutes, until all the cauliflower is very soft and golden brown in spots. Remove from the pan and allow to cool for about 10 minutes (enough to handle without burning your fingers).

Peel the garlic cloves and place the soft, roasted garlic in the bowl of a food processor along with the cauliflower and any oil that's pooled in the pan (there may not be any; that's fine) along with the beans and tahini. Process (in batches, if necessary), until you have a thick, smooth mixture. If the mixture is too dry, add the extra olive oil at this point.

Scrape the mixture into a bowl and sprinkle with salt and pepper; taste and adjust the seasonings. Serve immediately. Will keep, covered in the refrigerator, for up to 4 days.

Sweet and Spicy Roasted Chickpeas
Good for: all stages

This roasted chickpea recipe is a great way to incorporate more protein and healthy fats into your day via one very addictive snack. If you prefer really crispy chickpeas, continue to cook them beyond the time listed here.

MAKES 2 CUPS (480 ML) CHICKPEAS

2 tablespoons (30 ml) tahini (sesame paste)
2 tablespoons (30 ml) extra-virgin olive oil, preferably organic
2 teaspoons (10 ml) mild curry powder
2 teaspoons (10 ml) ground cinnamon
1 teaspoon (5 ml) Chinese 5-spice powder (see tip), or ½ teaspoon
    (2.5 ml) each ground cinnamon and ground ginger
Pinch of cayenne pepper, or to taste
⅛ teaspoon (0.5 ml) fine sea salt
10 drops plain or vanilla pure liquid stevia
2 cups (240 ml) well-cooked chickpeas, rinsed and drained.

Preheat the oven to 350°F (180°C). Line a rimmed cookie sheet with parchment.

In a medium-size bowl, whisk together all the ingredients, except the chickpeas, until smooth. Add the chickpeas to the bowl and gently fold over and over until they are well coated. Transfer to the prepared cookie sheet and spread out in a single layer. If any coating is left in the bowl, drizzle it evenly over the chickpeas.

Bake for 30 minutes, then remove from the oven and gently stir the chickpeas to redistribute. Bake for another 15 to 25 minutes, until the coating is dried and crispy in places. Allow to cool. Will keep, covered in the refrigerator, for up to 3 days.

Note: Chinese 5-spice powder is an aromatic combination of cinnamon, cloves, fennel, star anise, and Sichuan peppercorns, often used in Chinese cuisine. These days, prepared 5-spice powders are available even in mainstream supermarkets, but, if you can't find it, the alternative combination of cinnamon and ginger works well in this recipe, too.

"Sour Cream and Onion" Kale Chips
Good for: all stages

Warning: These chips are addictive! Luckily, they are a nutritious snack that just happens to deliver a serving of your daily leafy greens. If you're not on the kale bandwagon just yet, these chips will be sure to change that.

MAKES 4 SNACK SERVINGS (OR, IN MY CASE, SOMETIMES JUST 2)

⅓ cup (45 to 55 g) macadamia nuts or raw cashews
⅓ cup (55 g) raw hemp seeds (hemp hearts)
½ large onion, coarsely chopped
⅛ teaspoon (0.5 ml) fine sea salt, or to taste
3 tablespoons (45 ml) freshly squeezed lemon juice
2 teaspoons (10 ml) raw apple cider vinegar
5 drops plain pure liquid stevia, or to taste
⅓ cup (80 ml) filtered water
1 large head curly kale, stems removed, washed, and dried

Preheat the oven to 180°F (85°C). (If your oven doesn't go that low, preheat at its lowest setting.) Line two large cookie sheets with parchment.

In a powerful food processor, blend everything, except the kale, until the mixture is perfectly smooth and creamy. It should be the texture of a thick pancake batter: thin enough to pour, but thick enough to stick to the kale leaves without dripping off them.

Place the leaves in a large bowl (if your bowl isn't big enough, divide into batches). There's no need to tear them into smaller pieces (I don't), unless you want really small kale chips.

Pour the blended mixture over the leaves and toss with clean hands until the leaves are evenly coated. If you see bare spots here and there, you can rub them with some of the liquid from other leaves, or scrape them along the sides of the bowl where the topping seems to cling. The aim is to coat all the leaves as evenly as possible on all sides.

Place the leaves in a single layer (or as much as possible) on the prepared cookie sheets. Bake for 1 hour, then remove from the oven and flip over the kale leaves to expose the undersides. Bake for another hour, then check for doneness. Remove any leaves that are perfectly dry and brittle and allow to cool; return the other chips to the oven and bake for another 20 minutes or so. Continue to remove the leaves as they are done, leaving the moist ones in the oven for 20-minute intervals, until all the chips are dry and crispy. Store in an airtight container at room temperature. Will keep, covered, for up to 1 week.

Note: If you have a dehydrator, you can dehydrate the chips instead at 115°F (46°C) for 8 to 10 hours, until dry and crisp.

Zucchini Chips
Good for: all stages

I never knew how much I liked zucchini until I created these chips! While the zucchini does shrink considerably when baked, it's worth the effort to slice a lot at once (and so much easier if you have a mandoline). Baking at a low temperature allows the zucchini's moisture to dry out and the chips to crisp up and caramelize a bit. Heavenly!

MAKES ABOUT 2 CUPS (480 ML) CHIPS

6 to 8 large zucchini, washed and ends trimmed
¼ cup (60 ml) extra-virgin olive oil, preferably organic
Fine sea salt

Preheat the oven to 200°F (93°C). Line four cookie sheets with parchment.

Using a mandoline or a very sharp knife, cut the zucchini into thin rounds (no more than ⅛ inch [3 mm] thick). Transfer the rounds to a large bowl and toss well with the oil until they are evenly coated.

Place the rounds in a single layer on the prepared cookie sheets and sprinkle with salt. Bake for 1 hour, then check to see whether any of the chips are dry and browned; remove those. Bake for another 30 minutes to 1 hour, checking every 30 minutes and removing any chips that are already done. Remove from the oven when the remainder of the chips are all lightly browned and dry. Allow to cool and enjoy. Will keep, covered at room temperature, for up to 3 days.

Raw Carrot Cake Energy Balls
Good for: all stages

Q&E

When you need an afternoon pick-me-up and find yourself craving something a little sweet, these carrot cake balls do the trick. I've deliberately made the recipe small here, to reduce the risk of overdoing it when a craving strikes.

MAKES 6 TO 8 BALLS

½ cup (70 g) raw sunflower seeds
¾ teaspoon (7.5 ml) ground cinnamon
¼ teaspoon (1 ml) grated fresh ginger, or ⅛ teaspoon (0.5 ml)
    ground
2 teaspoons (10 ml) lemon zest
1 teaspoon (5 ml) ground flaxseeds
1/16 teaspoon (0.5 ml) stevia powder, or ¼ teaspoon (1 ml) plain
    or lemon-flavored pure liquid stevia (about 20 drops)
1 tablespoon (15 ml) unsweetened shredded coconut, plus
    more for rolling (optional)
½ teaspoon (2.5 ml) freshly squeezed lemon juice
1 teaspoon (5 ml) yacon syrup
1 teaspoon (5 ml) water
3 tablespoons (45 ml) finely grated carrot

In the bowl of a food processor, process the sunflower seeds, cinnamon, ginger, lemon zest, flax, and stevia until powdered. Add the coconut, lemon juice, yacon syrup, and water and process until it comes together in a dough. Add the carrot and pulse to incorporate evenly.

Form into balls and roll in additional shredded coconut, if desired. Refrigerate until firm.

Note: For later stages of the diet, you can replace the yacon syrup with coconut nectar.

"Chocolate" Cookie Dough Truffle Balls
Good for: all stages

Q&E

This is another great cravings-kicker for those on early stages of the diet (for later stages, add cacao nibs for extra decadence). You can keep extra dough balls in the freezer for when you really need a treat.

MAKES 6 BALLS

¼ cup (30 g) raw walnuts
2 tablespoons (30 ml) raw sunflower seeds
1 tablespoon (15 ml) coconut flour
2 teaspoons (10 ml) ground flaxseeds
2 teaspoons (10 ml) carob powder
1/16 teaspoon (0.25 ml) pure stevia powder, or ⅛ teaspoon
    (0.5 ml) plain, vanilla, or chocolate-flavored pure liquid
    stevia
Fine sea salt
1 teaspoon (5 ml) coconut oil
1 teaspoon (5 ml) pure vanilla extract
2 teaspoons (10 ml) filtered water
1 teaspoon (5 ml) cacao nibs (optional, for later stages of the
    diet)

Using a food processor, grind the walnuts, sunflower seeds, flour, flax, carob powder, stevia, and salt to a powder. Add the coconut oil, vanilla, and water and process until it comes together in a ball. Add the nibs, if using, and pulse to incorporate. Form into small balls. Refrigerate until ready to eat.

CHAPTER 10

Soups, Sandwiches, and Spreads

Curried Carrot-Lentil Soup
Good for: all stages

While on the hunt for a quick and easy dinner one evening, I decided to combine most of the vegetables left in the refrigerator with red lentils to create this soup. My husband and I were both delighted with how flavorful and delicious the soup turned out, given the list of common ingredients from which it's made. As a bonus, it also cooks up quite quickly because of the red lentils. This was a favorite recipe among the book's testers, too.

MAKES 4 SERVINGS

2 tablespoons (30 ml) extra-virgin olive oil, preferably organic
1 medium-size onion, chopped
3 garlic cloves, finely chopped
2 celery stalks, diced
5 medium-size carrots, diced
1 tablespoon (15 ml) mild curry powder
1 teaspoon (5 ml) ground cumin

145

1 teaspoon (5 ml) freshly squeezed lemon juice
Fine sea salt and freshly ground black pepper
1 cup (175 g) dried red lentils
½ cup (120 ml) chopped fresh cilantro or parsley leaves
4 cups (1 L) vegetable broth or stock
2 cups (480 ml) filtered water

In a large pot, heat the oil over medium heat. Add the onion, garlic, celery, and carrots and cook until the onion is translucent, for 7 to 10 minutes. Add the spices, lemon juice, salt and pepper to taste, and the lentils and cook for another minute.

Add the cilantro, broth, and water and increase the heat until the mixture comes to a boil; lower the heat to medium-low and cook, stirring occasionally, until the vegetables and lentils are soft, for about 30 minutes. Taste to adjust the seasonings and serve. May be frozen.

Q&E

Vegetable Miso Soup
Good for: all stages

When my husband and I were first together, I used to meet him at a sushi restaurant for lunch once a week near his office. It was during those lunches that I first learned to love miso soup. This version is definitely not traditional but is no less appealing with its complement of vegetables and cilantro. And it offers a speedy prep time. Be sure not to boil the miso, as that destroys the natural enzymes it contains. For a full light meal, add some Grain-Free Sandwich Bread (page 102) and you're all set.

MAKES 4 SERVINGS

⅓ cup (80 ml) unpacked dried arame (see tip)
1 cup (240 ml) warm filtered water
2 teaspoons (10 ml) extra-virgin olive oil
2 garlic cloves, sliced
2 medium-size carrots, peeled and cut into matchsticks

3 cups (720 ml) water

3 cups (720 ml) vegetable broth or stock

4 chard leaves, stems removed, cut into thin strips

3 tablespoons (45 ml) light or yellow miso

3 tablespoons (45 ml) coarsely chopped fresh cilantro leaves

In a small bowl, cover the arame with the warm water and set aside.

Heat the oil in the bottom of a soup pot and add the garlic and carrots. Sauté until the carrots begin to soften, for about 5 minutes. Add the water, broth, and chard and bring to a boil; simmer for another 5 minutes.

Meanwhile, in a small bowl, mix the miso with about ¼ cup (60 ml) of the broth from the pot. Once the soup is ready, turn off the heat; pour the miso mixture into the pot and stir to combine. Drain the arame. Ladle the soup into four soup bowls and sprinkle each with about one quarter each of the arame and the cilantro. Serve.

Tip: Although it resembles black spaghetti when wet, dried arame (as it's sold) is light and somewhat fragile. When measuring, you want to set it lightly in the measuring cup, allowing the air spaces between threads to remain. Packing it will result in much more arame than you'll need! While it's not an exact science, handling your arame gently before soaking will prevent any huge discrepancies in the final amount.

Roasted Garlic and Cauliflower Soup with Herbed Dumplings
Good for: all stages

If you're not a fan of cauliflower on its own, you may become a convert once you take a spoonful of this silky, smooth soup. The coconut milk adds both richness and density, while the roasted garlic provides a depth of flavor and slight umami kick that, together, is totally irresistible. The dumplings are divine, but the soup is great without them, too.

MAKES 4 TO 6 GENEROUS SERVINGS

1 whole head garlic, papery skin and cloves intact
1 tablespoon plus 1 teaspoon (20 ml) extra-virgin olive oil,
    preferably organic
1 large onion, chopped
1 medium-size cauliflower, trimmed and cut into florets
5 cups (1,200 ml) vegetable broth or stock
1 cup (240 ml) canned full-fat coconut milk
¼ teaspoon (1 ml) ground thyme
1 teaspoon (5 ml) freshly squeezed lemon juice
Fine sea salt and freshly ground pepper
Herbed Dumplings (optional; see note)

Bake the garlic: Preheat the oven to 375°F (190°C). Cut across the top of the head of the garlic to expose a bit of each clove. Drizzle with 1 teaspoon (5 ml) of the olive oil. Wrap in foil and bake until the cloves are all soft and golden, for about 40 minutes.

Meanwhile, prepare the rest of the soup: In a large pot or Dutch oven, heat the remaining table-spoon (15 ml) of oil over medium heat. Add the onion and sauté until translucent, for 8 to 10 minutes. Add the cauliflower, broth, coconut milk, and thyme and bring to a boil. Lower the heat, cover, and simmer until the cauliflower is soft, for 20 to 30 minutes.

Once the cauliflower is soft and the garlic is cool enough to handle, hold the garlic with the root end up over the pot and squeeze the bottom so that the cloves are squeezed out into the soup. Add the lemon juice and salt and pepper to taste. Allow to cool for about 5 minutes.

Blend the soup in batches in a blender until perfectly smooth. Return the pureed soup to the pot and adjust the seasonings. Bring the heat to a low simmer and cook until heated through. Serve. May be frozen.

Note: For the dumplings, use the recipe for Herbed Grain-Free Gnocchi (page 188), but use only 1 cup (160 g) of flour. Mix as for gnocchi, leaving the dough in the bowl instead of rolling it out (note that this dough will be much more like a muffin batter than a regular dough; this is fine). Drop the dough by teaspoonfuls (about 5 ml) into the soup, continuing until all the dough is used. Allow to simmer for 5 to 10 extra minutes, until the dumplings have expanded a bit and are cooked through. Serve.

Q&E

Quick and Easy Chard and Chickpea Soup
Good for: all stages

Yes, you can have home-cooked soup in a jiffy, even on a weeknight. Pair a bowl of this soup with a slice of Grain-Free Sandwich Bread (page 102) and some almond butter for a full meal.

MAKES 6 SERVINGS

1 tablespoon (15 ml) virgin coconut oil or extra-virgin olive oil, preferably organic

1 large onion, chopped

2 garlic cloves, chopped

1 bunch chard (6 to 8 leaves), stems removed and chopped, leaves shredded (2 to 3 cups [480 to 720 ml] leaves)

4 cups (1 L) vegetable broth or stock (homemade or use organic with no sugar or additives)

3 cups (720 ml) canned diced tomatoes

2 cups (480 ml) cooked chickpeas, drained

1 teaspoon (5 ml) dried oregano

2 teaspoons (10 ml) dried basil, or ¼ cup [60 ml] fresh

½ teaspoon (2.5 ml) onion salt

¼ cup (60 ml) chopped fresh parsley

½ teaspoon (2.5 ml) fine sea salt, or to taste

1 teaspoon (5 ml) freshly squeezed lemon juice

In a large pot or Dutch oven, heat the oil over medium heat and add the onion and garlic. Sauté until the onion is translucent, for about 8 minutes. Add the remaining ingredients, except the lemon juice, and bring to a light boil. Lower the heat to a simmer, cover, and simmer until all the vegetables are soft and the flavors are well combined, for about 30 minutes. Add the lemon juice; stir and adjust the seasonings. Serve. May be frozen.

Creamy Broccoli Soup
Good for: all stages

Q&E

This easy soup gets its creamy texture from an unlikely source—raw walnuts! Unlike cashews, walnuts add an earthy, robust flavor to the soup, making it perfect for winter dinners. The soup cooks up quickly and makes a great first course for a hearty kale salad (see pages 170 and 172) or some Herbed Grain-Free Gnocchi (page 188).

MAKES 4 TO 6 SERVINGS

1 tablespoon (15 ml) extra-virgin olive oil, preferably organic
1 medium-size onion, chopped
½ cup (55 g) raw walnut halves or pieces
2 garlic cloves, minced
1 medium-size head broccoli, woody ends removed (stems are
    fine), trimmed and chopped (about 4 cups [1 L] broccoli)
¼ cup (60 ml) chopped fresh dill, or 2 tablespoons (30 ml)
    dried (I recommend fresh for best flavor, if you can get it)
1 tablespoon (15 ml) mild miso
Fine sea salt
4 cups (1 L) vegetable broth or stock
2 teaspoons (10 ml) freshly squeezed lemon juice

In a large pot or Dutch oven, heat the oil over medium heat and add the onion and walnuts. Cook, stirring frequently, until the onion is translucent and the walnuts have begun to brown, for 8 to 10 minutes. Add the garlic and cook for 1 more minute. Add the remaining ingredients, except for the lemon juice, and stir well. Bring to a boil, then lower the heat to a simmer, cover, and cook until the broccoli is soft, for 10 to 15 minutes. Turn off the heat and allow the soup to cool somewhat.

Transfer the mixture to a blender, in batches if necessary, and blend until silky smooth (an immersion blender will leave a lot of texture to the soup, which may not be as pleasant to eat). Return the soup to the pot if necessary to warm it through, for 5 to 10 minutes. Add the lemon juice and stir to combine. Serve. May be frozen.

The "Toronto" Sandwich
Good for: all stages

Q&E

I decided to name this dish in honor of my favorite Canadian city. Because the wrapper can be whipped up in less than 10 minutes, I often make one of these for a quick, savory, weekday breakfast if I have leftover salad or cooked vegetables to stuff inside. If you have more time, try a "Toronto" Sandwich for Sunday brunch, filled with Glazed Tempeh (page 111) and your choice of vegetables. Don't forget the sauerkraut, though—it really makes the dish!

MAKES 1 SANDWICH

Wrapper
¼ cup (25 g) chickpea flour
Pinch of fine sea salt
3 to 4 tablespoons (45 to 60 ml) vegetable broth or stock
Nonstick spray, or olive or coconut oil, for pan

Filling Base
2 to 3 slices baked Glazed Tempeh (page 111) (optional)
2 to 3 tablespoons (30 to 45 ml) well-drained sauerkraut,
    preferably homemade (page 109) or kimchi
Handful of shredded lettuce or salad greens, or leftover cooked
    vegetables (e.g., the Creamy Greens with Asian Seasonings,
    page 174)

Creamy Topper
½ avocado, peeled, pitted, and sliced, ¼ cup (60 ml) hummus,
    or ¼ cup (60 ml) creamy dip of choice (e.g., the Savory
    Almond Sauce, page 178; Fresh Spicy Tomato Dressing or
    Sauce, page 180; or Tangy Cashew Cheese, page 158)

Make the wrapper: In a small bowl, whisk together the chickpea flour and salt. Add the broth and whisk until smooth and pourable but not watery (like pancake batter). If it's too thin, add a bit more flour; if too thick, add a touch more broth.

Grease a 6- to 8-inch (15 to 20 cm) skillet with nonstick spray, or brush with a little olive or coconut oil and heat over medium heat. Add the wrapper batter, spreading out to coat the pan, if necessary, and allow to cook until the top appears dry and the color has darkened, for 5 to 7 minutes. Flip and continue to cook for another 3 to 4 minutes on the other side.

While the wrapper cooks, prepare the fillings: Heat the tempeh, if using, in a nonstick pan and set aside. Drain the sauerkraut and set aside. If using lettuce, chop it now.

Assemble the sandwich: Once the wrapper is cooked, top half of it with the tempeh; then the greens and sauerkraut. Finally, add the avocado or drizzle with your choice of a creamy topper. Fold the wrapper over the fillings and consume immediately.

Spicy Beans with Chickpea Flatbreads
Good for: all stages

(Q&E)

This makes a great lunch or dinner. But it's also a terrific breakfast: one of the best ways to overcome cravings, as I mentioned in Chapter 4, is to start the day on a savory note—and this is one of my favorite savory breakfasts. Either black or kidney beans work well here; in later stages, you can also use fava beans.

MAKES 4 SERVINGS

Beans
2 tablespoons (30 ml) extra-virgin olive oil, preferably organic
1 medium-size onion, diced
3 garlic cloves, minced
½ to 1 small jalapeño pepper, coarsely chopped
1 small tomato, diced (optional)
½ teaspoon (2.5 ml) dried cumin
Fine sea salt and freshly ground black pepper
½ cup (120 ml) vegetable broth or stock
1½ cups (360 ml) well-cooked black, navy, or kidney beans,
    well drained (they should be very soft)
Up to 2 cups (480 ml) greens of choice, shredded (I like a mix of
    collards and kale)
2 green onions, thinly sliced, for garnish (optional)

Flatbreads (makes 4 flatbreads)
1 cup (100 g) chickpea flour
½ teaspoon (2.5 ml) ground cumin (optional)
¼ teaspoon (1 ml) fine sea salt
⅔ to 1 cup (160 to 240 ml) vegetable broth
1 tablespoon (15 ml) extra-virgin olive oil, preferably organic
2 tablespoons (30 ml) freshly squeezed lemon juice

Prepare the beans: Heat the oil in a large skillet over medium-high heat and add the onion and garlic. Sauté for 5 to 7 minutes, until the onion is translucent. Add the jalapeño and tomato, if using, and fry for another couple of minutes. Add the remaining ingredients, except for the greens and green onions, and stir well. Using the back of a spoon, mash the beans here and there so that about half the beans are mashed (leave some whole). Add the greens, if using. Lower to simmer, cover, and cook while you prepare the flatbread. Stir occasionally and add more broth if the mixture is too dry (it should be moist but not watery).

Make the flatbreads: Sift together the chickpea flour, cumin, and salt. In a measuring cup, mix together ⅔ cup (80 ml) of the broth with the oil and lemon juice. Pour the liquid over the dry ingredients and stir quickly to combine. The texture should be that of a loose pancake batter. If it's too thick, add up to ⅓ cup (80 ml) more broth as necessary.

Heat a nonstick skillet over medium heat. Using about ½ cup (120 ml) of batter for each flatbread, pour the mixture into the pan and swirl around to cover the bottom of the pan evenly (I find that using the back of a soup ladle really helps distribute it easily). It should begin to bubble a bit. Allow to cook undisturbed for 4 to 6 minutes, until the top is darker, dry, and the edges begin to brown. Gently flip and cook for another 1 to 2 minutes. Slide onto a plate and keep warm as you complete the flatbreads.

To serve: Scoop about one quarter of the bean mixture onto a pancake and sprinkle with the green onions. Will keep, covered (wrap the flatbreads in plastic) in the fridge, for up to 3 days.

Q&E

Chocolate Bean Butter
Good for: all stages

I love chocolate-based nut butters, but I don't always want to consume that much fat. I decided that combining cacao and beans with coconut oil provided an equally alluring spread, but one that provided an extra kick of protein in addition to less fat per serving! When blended together this way, the beans become smooth and creamy, lending the spread a bit of substance without conferring a "beany" flavor. It's one of my favorite snack spreads.

MAKES ABOUT 2 CUPS (480 ML) BEAN BUTTER

1 (19-ounce [540 ml]) can black beans, drained and rinsed, or
    2 cups (480 ml) well-cooked and drained beans
5 tablespoons (35 g) raw cacao powder (see note)
¼ cup (60 ml) yacon syrup
¼ teaspoon (1 ml) stevia powder, or 40 to 50 drops plain or
    vanilla pure liquid stevia, or to taste
Pinch of fine sea salt
3 tablespoons (45 ml) unrefined coconut oil, preferably organic

1 teaspoon (5 ml) pure vanilla extract
Up to 2 tablespoons (30 ml) water or unsweetened almond
    milk, if needed

Place all the ingredients in the bowl of a food processor and process until perfectly smooth, scraping down the sides as necessary. Once you think it's smooth, process for another minute. Spread on Grain-Free Sandwich Bread (page 102) or melt over Fluffy Pancakes (page 120) or ACD Whole-Grain Waffles (page 119). Scrape into a container or jar and store, covered, in the refrigerator for up to 3 days.

Note: If you find that cacao triggers cravings, you can make this spread with carob powder instead; increase the coconut oil to 4 tablespoons (60 ml).

High-Protein Carob-Hazelnut Butter
Q&E
Good for: all stages

This spread is reminiscent of Nutella but uses carob instead of cocoa for those in early stages of the ACD. If you're comfortable with raw cacao, try that instead, or use a combination of the two. This spread is perfect over pancakes or waffles, or stir some into your morning Baked Quinoa Porridge or Pudding (page 126) or Almost Instant Grain-Free Breakfast Porridge (page 127) for an extra-creamy, chocolaty treat!

MAKES 2½ CUPS (600 ML) NUT BUTTER

4 cups (580 g) lightly toasted hazelnuts
3 tablespoons (45 ml) carob powder
¼ cup (60 ml) coconut oil, preferably organic
Pinch of fine sea salt
½ teaspoon (2.5 ml) plain or flavored pure liquid stevia (I used
    hazelnut flavor) (about 40 drops)
3 tablespoons (45 ml) plain pea protein powder (the only
    ingredient should be pea protein; you can use another
    protein if it's a single-ingredient protein, too)

In the bowl of a food processor, blend the hazelnuts until they break down to a thick nut butter. This will take 5 to 10 minutes, depending on the processor you have (and only 2 to 3 minutes if you use a high-speed blender). Add the carob, oil, salt, and stevia and blend until smooth and liquefied, another minute or two. Add the protein powder and process to incorporate. Pour into a clean jar and store in the refrigerator. Will keep, covered, for up to 2 weeks.

Note: If you don't have a high-speed blender but prefer a smoother nut butter, first prepare the recipe in a food processor, then transfer the softened nut butter to a blender in small batches and blend until liquefied.

Mexican Chocolate Sunflower Butter
Good for: all stages

Q&E

Stevia and chocolate can be a tricky pairing, as some people find that the stevia brings out the bitterness in the chocolate. To mitigate this effect, I always use the bare minimum of stevia necessary to achieve an acceptable level of sweetness. This spread is delicious drizzled over Fluffy Pancakes (page 120) or ACD Whole-Grain Waffles (page 119). I also like it slathered on a piece of toasted Grain-Free Sandwich Bread (page 102)

MAKES ABOUT 1 ¼ CUPS (300 ML) SUNFLOWER SEED BUTTER

2 cups (280 g) lightly toasted sunflower seeds
5 tablespoons (40 g) raw cacao powder (see note)
5 tablespoons (75 ml) coconut oil, preferably organic
⅛ teaspoon (0.5 ml) fine sea salt, or to taste
1 tablespoon (15 ml) ground cinnamon, or to taste
Pinch of cayenne pepper, or to taste
1 teaspoon (5 ml) vanilla or chocolate-flavored pure liquid
   stevia (e.g., NuNaturals or SweetLeaf)
¼ cup (60 ml) yacon syrup
⅛ teaspoon (0.5 ml) pure stevia powder or more liquid stevia,
   or to taste
2 teaspoons (10 ml) pure vanilla extract

In the bowl of a food processor, blend the seeds until they break down to small crumbs for 2 to 3 minutes (about 30 seconds in a high-speed blender). Add the cacao and continue to process until almost powdered, then add the coconut oil and blend until perfectly smooth and liquefied, up to 5 minutes. (If using a high-speed blender with a tamper, this will take about 5 minutes total.) Add the remaining ingredients and blend to combine. Store in a clear jar in the refrigerator for up to 2 weeks.

Note: If you find that cacao triggers cravings, you can make this spread with carob powder instead; increase the coconut oil to 6 tablespoons (90 ml).

Gingerbread Pecan Butter
Good for: all stages

Q&E

Like gingerbread—but spreadable! As pecans can be expensive, feel free to use walnuts or almonds instead. The result is equally irresistible.

MAKES ABOUT 2 CUPS (500 ML) PECAN BUTTER

2 cups (225 g) lightly toasted pecan pieces
2 tablespoons (30 ml) coconut oil, preferably organic
2 teaspoons (10 ml) ground cinnamon
½ teaspoon (2.5 ml) ground ginger
Pinch of cloves
2 tablespoons (30 ml) yacon syrup
Plain or vanilla pure liquid stevia (I use about 15 drops)

In the bowl of a food processor, blend the pecans until they form crumbs that resemble bread crumbs. Continue to process, scraping the sides as necessary, until they break down to a nut butter consistency. Add the coconut oil and continue to process until the mixture liquefies.

Add the remaining ingredients and blend until well combined (it will thicken somewhat, but should still remain spreadable). Pour into a clean pint-size (500 ml) jar and store, covered in the refrigerator, for up to 2 weeks.

Coconut-Cranberry Spread
Good for: all stages

Q&E

A cross between a jam and coconut butter, this delightful spread is quick and easy to make. Use it on pancakes, waffles, toast, or in the Protein-Boost Cranberry Smoothie (page 116). And the vibrant pink color will bring a smile to anyone's face!

MAKES 2 CUPS (480 ML) SPREAD

1 recipe Festive Cranberry Sauce (page 182), at room
    temperature or warm
1 cup (240 ml) melted Homemade Coconut Butter (page 100)
Stevia

In a bowl, combine the cranberry sauce with the coconut butter, and stevia to taste until smooth and creamy. Transfer to a clean jar and store in the refrigerator. Will keep, covered in the refrigerator, for up to 2 weeks.

Tangy Cashew Cheese
Good for: all stages

This cashew cheese will surprise you with its rich, creamy texture and tangy flavor, reminiscent of those small wax-coated rounds of cheese that come wrapped in red mesh bags in the supermarket. If you're feeling adventurous, use the sauerkraut juice option, which will add a good dose of probiotics to the mix. Otherwise, raw apple cider vinegar works well, too.

MAKES ABOUT 2 CUPS (480 ML) CHEESE

2 cups (320 g) unsoaked raw cashews
3 tablespoons (45 ml) freshly squeezed lemon juice
1 tablespoon (15 ml) raw apple cider vinegar, or 2 to 3
    tablespoons (30 to 45 ml) juice from raw, lacto-fermented
    sauerkraut, or to taste

1½ tablespoons (22.5 ml) white or mellow miso

⅛ to ¼ teaspoon (0.5 to 1 ml) fine sea salt, or to taste

6 to 8 tablespoons (90 to 120 ml) filtered water (use more if
   necessary to blend)

Combine all the ingredients in a high-speed blender and blend, using the tamper to push the contents into the blades, until completely smooth. If desired, cover with plastic wrap and allow to ferment further at room temperature for up to 6 hours. Spread on crackers, bread, and so on.

Chunky Black Bean Spread
Q&E
Good for: all stages

Although I love cooking, for the most part, I'm a fairly lazy cook: if it takes too much fussing or a lot of chopping, I look for a quicker alternative (such as asking my hubby, the perfect sous-chef, to take care of that task). This simple spread provides a great flavor punch and makes a great filling for sandwiches or raw collard rolls, or as a dip with crackers or raw veggies. Because it's also ready in minutes without much effort, it may just be the ideal spread.

MAKES ABOUT 3 CUPS (720 ML) SPREAD

2 cups (480 ml) cooked or canned black beans, drained and
   rinsed

2 garlic cloves, minced

2 tablespoons (30 ml) smooth natural almond butter,
   sunflower seed butter, or tahini (sesame paste)

¼ cup (60 ml) chopped fresh cilantro or parsley

1 tablespoon (15 ml) freshly squeezed lemon juice

⅔ cup (160 ml) chopped tomatoes (I used grape tomatoes)

2 green onions, chopped

Fine sea salt and freshly ground black pepper

In the bowl of a food processor, combine 1½ cups (360 ml) of the beans with the garlic, almond butter, cilantro, and lemon juice. Process until smooth. Add the remaining beans and pulse once or twice to chop them up. Turn the mixture into a bowl and stir in the tomatoes and green onions. Season to taste. Serve with raw carrots, pepper chunks, celery sticks, or other veggies, or use as the filling for a raw collard roll or sandwich on Grain-Free Sandwich Bread (page 102).

Raw Almond-Veggie Pâté
Good for: all stages

I first encountered raw veggie pâtés when I took a series of raw food classes while in nutrition school and immediately fell in love with the flavors of soaked almonds pureed with raw veggies. Once soaked, the almonds become milder, smoother, and softer—perfect for blending into a creamy spread that works on all kinds of crackers or as a dip for even more veggies.

MAKES 10 TO 15 APPETIZER SERVINGS

1 cup (170 g) raw natural almonds, soaked in room-
    temperature, filtered water for 6 to 10 hours and drained
½ cup (70 g) raw pumpkin seeds, soaked in room-temperature,
    filtered water for 4 to 6 hours and drained
1 medium-size carrot, peeled and cut into chunks
½ cup (120 ml) coarsely chopped broccoli
½ red bell pepper, cored and cut into chunks
½ medium-size ripe tomato, cut into chunks
1 large garlic clove, sliced
½ cup (120 ml) fresh cilantro (leaves and thin stems), or to
    taste
2 tablespoons (30 ml) white or mild miso paste
2 to 3 tablespoons (30 to 45 ml) freshly squeezed lemon juice
Fine sea salt and freshly ground black pepper

In the bowl of a food processor, process the soaked almonds, soaked pumpkin seeds, and carrot until well ground. Add the remaining ingredients and continue to process, stopping to scrape down the sides of the bowl occasionally, until you have a smooth paste. (Add more lemon juice, miso, or water, if necessary, to achieve your desired texture.) Season to taste.

Scrape the pâté into a serving bowl and chill until ready to spread on crackers or serve with crudités. Store in refrigerator for up to 5 days.

My Favorite Hummus
Good for: all stages

Q&E

Hummus is a classic dip and a regular source of protein on vegan diets. While most hummus contains quite a bit of oil, I discovered a few years ago that I prefer mine a bit thicker and creamier, with a touch of almond butter added to the tahini. The result is one delicious, oil-free spread or dip. (If you prefer to avoid nuts, you can substitute sunflower butter or olive oil for the almonds, of course.)

MAKES ABOUT 2 CUPS (480 ML) HUMMUS

2 cups (480 ml) cooked, rinsed, and well-drained chickpeas
Juice of ½ lemon (about 2 tablespoons [30 ml])
2 garlic cloves, minced
½ teaspoon (2.5 ml) ground cumin
½ teaspoon (2.5 ml) smoked paprika
2 heaping tablespoons (40 ml) smooth natural almond butter
3 heaping tablespoons (55 ml) tahini (sesame paste)
⅓ cup (80 ml) chopped fresh parsley
Fine sea salt
Water, as needed, up to ¼ cup (60 ml)

Combine all the ingredients in the bowl of a food processor and blend until smooth. If the hummus is too thick, add water and continue to blend until smooth and creamy. Taste and adjust the seasonings. Store, covered, in the refrigerator for up to 3 days.

CHAPTER 11

Salads, Dressings, and Sauces

Cabbage and Broccoli Slaw
Good for: all stages

Q&E

Cabbage and broccoli make a perfect pair in this crunchy, colorful slaw. I'm a huge fan of fresh dill in coleslaw, which screams "summer" to me, any time of year, but, if you're not a fan, feel free to swap it out for chopped parsley or another fresh herb of choice instead. This salad works well alongside almost any main dish.

MAKES 4 TO 5 SIDE SALAD SERVINGS

Salad
2 cups (480 ml) finely shredded red or green cabbage
2 cups (480 ml) broccoli florets
2 green onions, chopped
½ red bell pepper, cored and diced (optional)
⅓ cup (50 g) raw pumpkin seeds
1 carrot, grated

Dressing
⅔ cup (90 to 110 g) raw macadamia nuts or cashews
6 tablespoons (90 ml) freshly squeezed lemon juice

2 tablespoons (30 ml) raw apple cider vinegar

1 teaspoon (5 ml) dry mustard

¾ teaspoon (3.5 ml) mild paprika

2 small garlic cloves, chopped

¼ cup (60 ml) chopped fresh dill, or 2 tablespoons (30 ml)
   dried dill or parsley

Fine sea salt

3 to 5 drops pure liquid stevia, or to taste

⅔ cup (160 ml) filtered water, or a bit more, as needed

Assemble the salad: Place all the salad ingredients in a bowl.

Prepare the dressing: In the bowl of a high-powered blender, combine all the dressing ingredients, including salt to taste, and blend until smooth. Pour the dressing over the salad and toss to coat.

Q&E

Crimson Salad
Good for: all stages

This vibrant, refreshing salad combines the brisk tang of lime with the natural sweetness of beets and carrots. Crunchy pecans and pumpkin seeds offer textural contrast and a protein boost. I love this salad any time of year but particularly enjoy it in spring when the colors herald the coming flowers blooming outside as well.

MAKES 4 SIDE SALAD SERVINGS

Salad
1 large beet, peeled (should be fresh and firm)

2 large carrots, peeled

½ cup (50 g) chopped pecans, lightly toasted

¼ cup (35 g) pumpkin seeds, lightly toasted

Dressing

1 garlic clove, minced

¼ cup (60 ml) freshly squeezed lime juice (about 2 limes)

¼ cup (60 ml) extra-virgin olive oil, preferably organic

3 tablespoons (45 ml) chopped fresh cilantro or parsley

Pinch of fine sea salt

3 to 5 drops plain pure liquid stevia, or to taste

Prepare the salad: Using the medium grater on a food processor, mandoline, or hand grater, grate the beets and carrots and place in a medium-size bowl with the nuts and the seeds. Set aside.

Make the dressing: In a small bowl, combine the dressing ingredients. Pour over the vegetable mixture and toss to coat everything well. Serve immediately. Will keep, refrigerated, for 2 days.

Q&E   Dandelion-Apple Salad
Good for: Stage 2 and beyond

This salad, with its tart, creamy dressing and coconut sprinkles, will remind you of a classic Waldorf. Dandelion is one of my favorite greens and a great superfood that supports effective liver function. If you find the dandelion too bitter on its own, you can use arugula or even chopped kale instead.

MAKES 4 SIDE SALAD SERVINGS

Dressing

1 medium-size sweet, crisp apple (e.g., Gala, Fuji, or Pink Lady)

¼ cup (60 ml) extra-virgin olive oil, preferably organic

2 tablespoons (30 ml) raw apple cider vinegar

2 tablespoons (30 ml) freshly squeezed lemon juice

¼ teaspoon (1 ml) dry mustard

1 large or 2 small garlic cloves

¼ teaspoon (1 ml) ground fennel seeds

5 to 8 drops plain pure liquid stevia, or to taste

Salad
1 bunch dandelion leaves, trimmed and chopped into 2-inch
    (5 cm) pieces; or use a combination of dandelion and baby
    greens
1 medium-size sweet, crisp apple (e.g., Gala, Fuji, or Pink
    Lady), cored and diced
2 medium-size carrots, grated
2 celery stalks, diced
⅓ cup (35 g) walnut pieces or halves, raw or lightly toasted
¼ cup (60 ml) unsweetened shredded coconut
¼ cup (60 ml) chopped fresh parsley leaves (optional)

Make the dressing: Core the apple and chop it into large pieces (if you have a strong blender, leave the skin on). Place in a blender with the remaining dressing ingredients and blend until smooth and creamy. If the dressing is too thick, add a tablespoon (15 ml) or two of water and blend until the desired thickness is achieved.

Make the salad: In a large bowl, combine the dandelion leaves with remaining the salad ingredients, except the coconut and parsley. Add the dressing and toss to coat. Sprinkle with the coconut and parsley and serve.

Fennel, Brussels Sprout, and Edamame Salad
Good for: all stages

This salad reminds me of *vinegret*, a Russian root vegetable salad mixed with fermented veggies. Roasted vegetables and sauerkraut may sound like an odd coupling, but the textures meld beautifully and the flavors really pop. Apart from roasting, this is a really simple dish to make.

MAKES 3 TO 4 SIDE SALAD SERVINGS OR 2 MAIN DISH SERVINGS

Coconut oil, for pan (optional)
1 large fennel bulb, trimmed and cut into thick slices
2 cups (480 mg) Brussels sprouts, trimmed and cut into quarters

2 tablespoons (30 ml) extra-virgin olive oil, preferably organic

½ teaspoon (2.5 ml) dried oregano

2 tablespoons (30 ml) raw apple cider vinegar

1 tablespoon (15 ml) freshly squeezed lemon juice

Fine sea salt and freshly ground black pepper

⅓ cup (80 ml) chopped fresh parsley

1 cup (240 ml) cooked, cooled shelled edamame

½ teaspoon (2.5 ml) whole caraway seeds (optional)

½ cup (120 ml) well-drained, naturally fermented sauerkraut
    (the kind you have to refrigerate)

Preheat the oven to 400°F (200°C). Line a large roasting pan with parchment, or grease lightly with coconut oil. Place the fennel and Brussels sprouts in the prepared pan and drizzle with 1 tablespoon (15 ml) of the olive oil. Toss to coat. Bake until the veggies are soft but not browned, for 20 to 30 minutes. Allow to cool to room temperature.

Meanwhile, in a large bowl, whisk together the remaining tablespoon (15 ml) of olive oil and the oregano, vinegar, and lemon juice. Taste and adjust the seasonings, if necessary. Add the salt, pepper, parsley, edamame, and caraway seeds.

Once the vegetables are cool, add them to the bowl along with the sauerkraut and toss everything together. Serve.

Baby Greens with Pear and Walnuts in Cranberry–Poppy Seed Dressing
Good for: Stage 2 and beyond

Q&E

Baby greens, toasted walnuts, pear, and goat cheese was one of my go-to recipes for entertaining. I've updated this classic so it's ACD-friendly. Both the tang and creaminess of the cheese is provided by the vibrantly crimson dressing, offering a lovely counterpart to the greens and pear. It's also a perfect way to use more of your homemade Festive Cranberry Sauce (page 182).

MAKES 4 SIDE SALAD SERVINGS

Dressing
½ cup (120 ml) Festive Cranberry Sauce (page 182)
2 tablespoons (30 ml) extra-virgin olive oil, preferably organic
Juice of ½ lime
2 teaspoons (10 ml) raw apple cider vinegar
1 tablespoon (15 ml) poppy seeds
⅓ to ½ cup (80 to 120 ml) water, as needed
Pinch of fine sea salt

Salad
About 6 cups (1.5 L) mixed baby greens (mesclun greens or a
    combination of baby kale, chard, spinach, arugula [rocket],
    etc.)
1 large pear, cored and diced
½ cup (55 g) walnut halves or pieces, lightly toasted

Make the dressing: Place all the ingredients in a blender and blend until smooth.

Make the salad: Place the salad ingredients in a large bowl and toss gently with the dressing. Serve.

Q&E

Asian Napa Cabbage Salad
Good for: all stages

Classic Asian seasonings meld beautifully in this fantastic salad that will please everyone. You'll find that the dressing is really the star here; as one of the testers remarked, "The boyfriend said he wants to eat this forever. . . . I think he'd eat a piece of cardboard if it were covered in the dressing." It also works well as a dip or even topping for Herbed Grain-Free Gnocchi (page 188).

MAKES 4 TO 6 SIDE SALAD SERVINGS

Dressing
¼ cup (60 ml) smooth natural almond butter

1 garlic clove, minced

1 teaspoon (5 ml) minced fresh ginger

10 drops plain pure liquid stevia, or to taste

2 tablespoons (30 ml) freshly squeezed lime juice

2 teaspoons (10 ml) sesame oil

2 tablespoons (30 ml) Bragg Liquid Aminos or wheat-free
    tamari

1 tablespoon (15 ml) apple cider vinegar

¼ cup (60 ml) filtered water

⅛ teaspoon (0.5 ml) red pepper flakes

Salad
1 small napa cabbage, trimmed and cut into shreds

1 medium-size carrot, grated

2 green onions, sliced

⅓ cup (80 ml) chopped natural almonds, raw or lightly toasted

2 tablespoons (30 ml) sesame seeds, raw or lightly toasted

Make the dressing: Blend all the ingredients together in a small bowl.

Make the salad: Place all the salad ingredients, except the sesame seeds, in a bowl and toss with the dressing. Sprinkle with the sesame seeds and serve.

Creamy Kale Salad with Black Beans and Sweet Potato
Good for: all stages

Kale really is the darling of the vegetable world! When raw, I find the flavor to be incredibly mild and appealing, but it does retain a hardy chewiness that way. When you chop the kale and then "massage" it (see instructions), part of the cell walls are broken down, resulting in the perfect salad consistency. The contrast between the crisp kale, smooth sweet potato, and hearty beans is a trio made in salad heaven.

MAKES 4 SIDE SALAD SERVINGS OR 2 MAIN COURSE SERVINGS

Dressing
½ cup (70 g) raw shelled hemp seeds (hemp hearts)
Pure liquid stevia (I used about 8 drops plain)
¼ to ½ cup (60 to 120 ml) water, as needed
1 garlic clove, sliced
Juice of ½ lemon (about 2 tablespoons [30 ml])
2 teaspoons (10 ml) raw apple cider vinegar
½ teaspoon (1 ml) dry mustard

Salad
1 medium-size head curly kale (6 to 9 leaves)
Up to ½ teaspoon (2.5 ml) fine sea salt
1 tablespoon (15 ml) of olive oil
1 large sweet potato, baked, cooled, peeled, and cut into cubes
1½ cups (360 ml) cooked black beans (canned, well-rinsed beans are fine)
2 green onions, sliced
¼ cup (60 ml) chopped fresh parsley
½ sweet red pepper, cored and chopped

Make the dressing: Combine all the ingredients in a high-speed blender, starting with ¼ cup (60 ml) of water, and blend until smooth. Add up to ¼ cup (60 ml) more water, if desired, for a thinner dressing (it should be thick and creamy, to stick to the kale).

Make the salad: First, soften the kale: Remove the kale leaves from the stems; discard the stems, then wash and dry the leaves. Stack the leaves, roll tightly (jelly-roll style), then cut thinly crosswise to create long, thin shreds. Chop the shreds into smaller pieces and place in a large salad bowl.

Sprinkle the kale with salt and drizzle with about 1 tablespoon (15 ml) of olive oil. Using clean hands, "massage" the kale, squeezing it and squishing it between your fingers, until it begins to darken and soften a bit (this breaks down the fibers in the leaves and renders them more easily digestible—but they will still retain a nice crunch).

Add the sweet potato, beans, green onions, parsley, and red pepper.

Top with the dressing and toss gently to coat evenly.

As-You-Like Kale Salad
Good for: all stages (see note)

Q&E

Kale is one of my favorite superfoods, chock-full of antioxidants that fight cancer, anti-inflammatory compounds, a slew of vitamins and minerals, and a good amount of fiber. And best of all, it tastes great! This salad is also infinitely adaptable, depending on which combination of veggies you choose from each category. I generally use whatever I've got in the refrigerator that day, and the result is always delicious. As long as you include the base, a few crunchy veggies, and some fresh herbs and nuts or seeds, the rest can be omitted if desired and you'll still end up with a yummy salad.

MAKES 6 TO 8 SIDE SALAD SERVINGS OR 3 TO 5 MAIN COURSE SERVINGS.

The Base
1 bunch (6 to 9 leaves) curly kale or Swiss chard, or a combination
Salt
1 tablespoon (15 ml) olive oil
1 cup (240 ml) mixed baby salad greens, bite-size romaine lettuce,
    bite-size butter lettuce, arugula (rocket), or a combination

Crunchy Veggies
1 medium-size carrot, grated
1 medium-size beet, grated
1 celery stalk, diced
½ red, yellow, or orange bell pepper, cored and diced

Fresh Herbs
½ cup (120 ml) of at least 2 types of coarsely chopped fresh
    herbs (my favorites are dill, basil, mint, flat-leaf parsley,
    and cilantro)

Nuts and/or Seeds
½ cup (120 ml) total of any combination of fresh nut pieces
    and seeds (my favorite combinations are walnuts or pecans
    and hemp seeds; walnuts or pecans and sunflower seeds;
    almonds and pumpkin seeds)

The Crucifers

2 cups (480 ml) total of any of the following (or any combination):

Finely shredded green or red cabbage

Broccoli

Cauliflower

Fruit (if allowed; otherwise, omit):

1 apple or pear, cored and diced; or 1 cup (240 ml) fresh blueberries or strawberries; or 1 avocado, peeled, pitted, and diced

Other Add-Ins (all of these are optional)

½ fennel bulb, sliced thinly

4 to 6 radishes, sliced into half-moons

⅓ cucumber, sliced into half-moons

Handful of grape or cherry tomatoes, cut in half

Handful of sprouts (my favorites are sunflower, pea, or alfalfa sprouts)

1 recipe Classic Oil and Lemon Dressing (page 176)

Make the base: Soften the kale: Remove the kale leaves from the stems; discard the stems, then wash and dry the leaves. Stack the leaves, roll tightly (jelly-roll style), then cut thinly crosswise to create long, thin shreds. Chop the shreds into smaller pieces and place in a large salad bowl.

Sprinkle the kale with salt and drizzle with about 1 tablespoon (15 ml) of olive oil. Using clean hands, "massage" the kale, squeezing it and squishing it between your fingers, until it begins to darken and soften a bit (this breaks down the fibers in the leaves and renders them more easily digestible—but they will still retain a nice crunch). If using chard, wash and chop it using the same method and add to the bowl (it doesn't need to be massaged).

Assemble the salad: Add the remaining salad ingredients to the bowl. Drizzle with the dressing, toss, and serve. Will keep, covered in the refrigerator, for up to 3 days (and will still remain crunchy!).

Note: For Stage 1 of the diet, omit the fruit. It will still taste yummy!

Creamy Greens with Asian Seasonings
Good for: all stages

Q&E

This is a quick, easy, and really delicious way to enjoy your greens. Because Bragg Liquid Aminos or tamari is already quite salty, I don't include additional salt, but feel free to season to taste, if you prefer a saltier dish.

MAKES 4 SERVINGS

4 to 6 large kale leaves, stems removed
4 to 6 large chard leaves, stems removed
1 tablespoon (15 ml) extra-virgin coconut oil, preferably organic
3 garlic cloves, chopped
1 tablespoon (15 ml) minced fresh ginger
1 cup (240 ml) canned full-fat coconut milk
1 tablespoon (15 ml) chickpea flour
2 tablespoons (30 ml) Bragg Liquid Aminos or wheat-free tamari
2 tablespoons (30 ml) sesame seeds

Lay the kale and chard leaves flat on a cutting board and roll up tightly, jelly-roll style. Cut the "roll" into thin slices (about ¼ inch [6 mm] wide), creating long shreds of the greens. Set aside.

Heat the oil in a large skillet over medium heat. Add the garlic, ginger, and shredded greens and cook, stirring frequently, until the vegetables have begun to wilt and are bright green.

Meanwhile, in a small bowl, whisk together the coconut milk, chickpea flour, and liquid aminos until smooth. Pour this mixture over the greens in the pan and stir to coat well. The sauce will thicken fairly quickly and should cling to the leaves. Cook for about 2 minutes, until heated through. Place the greens on a platter and sprinkle with sesame seeds to serve.

Caesar Salad
Good for: all stages

One of the few things I missed when I first started the ACD was a good Caesar salad. This version is creamy, garlicky, and topped with vegan bacon and croutons. What's left to miss?

MAKES 4 SIDE SALAD SERVINGS OR 2 MAIN COURSE SERVINGS

Dressing
½ medium-size just-ripe avocado, peeled, pitted, and cut into
    chunks
1 garlic clove, chopped
2 teaspoons (10 ml) raw apple cider vinegar
2 tablespoons (30 ml) freshly squeezed lemon juice (about ½
    lemon)
1 teaspoon (5 ml) Bragg Liquid Aminos or wheat-free tamari
½ teaspoon (2.5 ml) dry mustard
2 tablespoons (30 ml) extra-virgin olive oil, preferably organic
1 to 5 drops plain pure liquid stevia
Pinch of fine sea salt
¼ to ⅓ (60 to 80 ml) water, as need to achieve desired
    consistency

Salad
1 medium-size head romaine lettuce, trimmed, cleaned, and
    torn into bite-size pieces
½ recipe Glazed Tempeh (page 111), crumbled
2 slices Grain-Free Sandwich Bread (page 102), cut into cubes
    and toasted on a cookie sheet at 350°F (180°C) until browned

Make the dressing: Blend all the ingredients in a high-powered blender until smooth and creamy. Taste and adjust the seasonings, if necessary.

Make the salad: Place the romaine in a salad bowl and toss well with the dressing. Sprinkle with the tempeh and croutons. Serve.

Classic Oil and Lemon Dressing
Good for: all stages

Q&E

This deceptively simple and flavorful dressing is a perfect accompaniment to any crisp, leafy green salad, or wherever you would have used a classic balsamic dressing. I also love it as a dip for freshly steamed artichokes.

MAKES ABOUT ⅓ CUP (80 ML) DRESSING

2 to 4 tablespoons (30 to 60 ml) extra-virgin olive oil,
    preferably organic
Juice of ½ large lemon
2 teaspoons (10 ml) raw apple cider vinegar
2 to 5 drops plain pure liquid stevia, or to taste
½ teaspoon (2.5 ml) dry mustard
Fine sea salt

Whisk all the ingredients together until emulsified; pour over the salad greens and toss. Store leftover dressing in a jar in the refrigerator for up to 5 days.

For Italian Dressing, add ½ teaspoon (2.5 ml) each of dried oregano and basil.

Cranberry–Poppy Seed Dressing
Good for: all stages

Q&E

I created this dressing as a way to use leftover Festive Cranberry Sauce (page 182) after our holiday feast. The flavor is rich and tart with just a hint of sweetness, perfect for salads made with raw bitter greens, such as arugula, dandelion, kale, or chard.

MAKES ABOUT 1 CUP (240 ML) DRESSING

½ cup (120 ml) Festive Cranberry Sauce (page 182)
2 tablespoons (30 ml) extra-virgin olive oil, preferably organic

Juice of ½ lime
2 teaspoons (10 ml) raw apple cider vinegar
1 tablespoon (15 ml) poppy seeds
⅓ to ½ cup (80 to 120 ml) water, as needed
Pinch of fine sea salt

Blend all the ingredients in a blender until smooth. Use on mild leafy greens. Store leftover dressing in a jar in the refrigerator for up to 3 days.

Perfect Golden Gravy
Good for: all stages

Q&E

If you're a fan of gravy with your holiday turkey, you'll recognize the deep golden hue of this gravy. Miso and Bragg Liquid Aminos add a savory, robust flavor that melds perfectly with the subtle smoky undertones from the paprika. My husband, who is very picky about what he'll pour over his mashed potatoes, adored this gravy with the Sunday Night Roast (page 196). It's also terrific over a slice of Grain-Free Sandwich Bread (page 102) for an ACD-friendly version of "biscuits" and gravy.

MAKES ABOUT 2 CUPS (480 ML) GRAVY

2 tablespoons (30 ml) white or mellow miso
1 cup (240 ml) well-cooked black-eyed peas, red kidney beans,
   fava beans, or other red or brown beans (see note)
1½ cups (360 ml) vegetable broth or stock
1½ tablespoons (22.5 ml) Bragg Liquid Aminos or wheat-free
   tamari
1 tablespoon (15 ml) extra-virgin olive oil, preferably organic
½ teaspoon (2.5 ml) dry mustard
½ teaspoon (2.5 ml) dried onion powder or onion salt
¼ teaspoon (1 ml) dried sage
½ teaspoon (2.5 ml) smoked paprika
1 garlic clove, chopped
1 tablespoon (15 ml) chickpea flour (optional)

Blend all the ingredients in a blender until smooth. Pour the mixture into a medium-size pot and cook over medium heat, stirring frequently to avoid scorching, until thickened, for 10 to 15 minutes. Use with Sunday Night Roast (page 196), mashed potatoes, fries, or wherever you like gravy! Store leftover gravy in a jar in the refrigerator for up to 3 days.

Note: Any kind of bean works here for a flavorful gravy, but, for a traditional "golden" color, you want red or brown beans; black beans will result in a somewhat gray and muddy-looking gravy, not nearly as appetizing!

Q&E   **Sweet or Savory Almond Sauce**
Good for: all stages

This sauce can be used two ways—sweet for topping Fluffy Pancakes (page 120) or drizzled on a baked sweet potato for a delicious, easy breakfast; or savory atop the Grain and Veggie Meal-in-a-Bowl (page 201), your favorite salad, or even as a sauce for Herbed Grain-Free Gnocchi (page 188). Because liquid aminos are quite salty, I don't add more salt to the savory version, but feel free to add some if you like.

MAKES ABOUT ⅓ CUP (80 ML) SAUCE

2 tablespoons (30 ml) smooth natural almond butter
1 teaspoon (5 ml) grated fresh ginger
½ teaspoon (2.5 ml) mild curry powder
½ teaspoon (2.5 ml) ground cinnamon
Up to 2 tablespoons (30 ml) water
Pinch of fine sea salt, or to taste

Plus: Sweet
10 drops plain or vanilla pure liquid stevia, or to taste
1 to 2 tablespoons (15 to 30 ml) unsweetened plain or vanilla
    almond, hemp, or Homemade Coconut Milk (page 99)

Plus: Savory
1 small garlic clove, minced

1 tablespoon (15 ml) Bragg Liquid Aminos or wheat-free tamari
Pinch of red pepper flakes

Combine all the ingredients, including your preference of sweet or savory additions, in a small bowl and whisk until smooth. Add milk (for sweet) or water (for savory), if necessary, to achieve your desired consistency.

Store, covered, in a jar in the refrigerator for up to 4 days.

Garlicky Warm Avocado Sauce
Q&E
Good for: all stages

A great accompaniment to Sunday Night Roast (page 196), this sauce is also delicious tossed with pasta, on top of the ACD Whole-Grain Waffles (page 119) for a light dinner, or as your sauce of choice in the Grain and Veggie Meal-in-a-Bowl (page 201). If left at room temperature, it's also lovely as a dip for raw veggies.

MAKES ABOUT 1 CUP (240 ML) SAUCE

1 medium-size just-ripe avocado, pitted and scooped from peel
¼ cup (60 ml) tahini (sesame paste)
1 teaspoon (5 ml) freshly squeezed lemon juice or raw apple
    cider vinegar
2 small garlic cloves, minced
1 teaspoon (5 ml) chopped fresh dill (optional), or chopped
    fresh cilantro or parsley
Up to 1 cup (240 ml) vegetable broth or stock
Salt

Combine all the ingredients in a food processor or blender, adding salt to taste, and blend until smooth. Transfer to a small pot and heat over medium-low heat, stirring constantly, until just warmed through. Use immediately. To prepare in advance as a cold dip, use less broth and refrigerate before using. Store by pressing a sheet of plastic wrap directly against the top of the dip to avoid contact with air. Use within 2 days.

Fresh Spicy Tomato Dressing or Sauce
Good for: all stages

Q&E

I love sriracha, the spicy-sweet chili sauce that's somewhat of a Thai version of ketchup, but it's a definite no-no on the ACD because of the sugar it contains. This quick and easy sauce reminded me of my beloved sriracha, with its deep red base, slight sweetness, and spiciness. Use it atop the Grain and Veggie Meal-in-a-Bowl (page 201), the Herbed Grain-Free Gnocchi (page 188), or any grains or salads. It's also great as a dip for raw vegetables.

MAKES ABOUT ½ CUP (120 ML) SAUCE

1 large tomato, chopped
1 garlic clove, minced
1 tablespoon (15 ml) raw apple cider vinegar
1 tablespoon (15 ml) Bragg Liquid Aminos or wheat-free
    tamari
⅓ cup (45 to 55 g) raw cashews or macadamia nuts
1 (1-inch [2.5 cm]) piece fresh ginger, peeled and grated
    (about 2 teaspoons [10 ml])
5 drops pure liquid stevia, or to taste
¼ to ½ teaspoon (1 to 2.5 ml) fine sea salt, or to taste
¼ teaspoon (1 ml) red pepper flakes, or to taste (optional)
Up to 3 tablespoons (45 ml) water, if necessary (optional)

Combine all the ingredients, except the water, in a high-powered blender and blend until smooth. If the sauce is too thick, add up to 3 tablespoons (45 ml) of water and blend again. Will keep in a closed container in the refrigerator for up to 3 days.

Broccoli-Lemon Pesto
Good for: all stages

Q&E

While not technically a "pesto" because it combines broccoli with the herbs and uses hemp seeds in place of pine nuts, this lovely puree is nevertheless a tasty, versatile spread that can be used wherever you'd use traditional pesto. I love this as a base for the Grain-Free Pizza Crust (page 104) or tossed with Herbed Grain-Free Gnocchi (page 188). It's also great as a sandwich spread or on crackers, to season soup or as a dip.

MAKES ABOUT ⅔ CUP (160 ML) PESTO

½ cup (120 ml) raw broccoli florets
⅓ cup (80 ml) fresh cilantro or parsley leaves
2 garlic cloves, coarsely chopped
¼ cup (60 ml) extra-virgin olive oil, preferably organic
Zest of 1 large lemon
Juice of ½ lemon (about 2 tablespoons [30 ml])
⅓ cup (50 g) raw shelled hemp seeds (hemp hearts)
¼ teaspoon fine sea salt
Up to 3 tablespoons (45 ml) water, if necessary (optional)

In the bowl of a food processor, blend all the ingredients, except the water, until smooth. If necessary, add up to 3 tablespoons (45 ml) of water to achieve your desired consistency. Will keep, covered, in the refrigerator up to 3 days; may be frozen.

Festive Cranberry Sauce
Good for: all stages

Q&E

Canned cranberry sauces may seem very convenient, but they are filled with sugar; this homemade version is healthier and can be made in a snap. I use any leftover cranberry sauce as a jam substitute on Grain-Free Sandwich Bread (page 102) or mixed into the Coconut-Cranberry Spread (page 158).

MAKES ABOUT 1 CUP (240 ML) SAUCE

2 cups (480 ml) fresh or frozen cranberries
2 tablespoons (30 ml) water
Zest of 1 lime or ½ large lemon (2 to 3 teaspoons [10 to 15 ml])
1 teaspoon (5 ml) pure vanilla extract
Small pinch of fine sea salt
Plain or flavored pure liquid stevia (I used about 40 drops of
    lemon-flavored, but I think you'd need less of the plain)

Place everything, except the stevia, in a small pot with a cover. Cover and bring to a boil over medium heat, then stir and lower the heat to a simmer. Cook, covered, stirring occasionally, until all the berries have popped and the sauce is thick, for 10 to 15 minutes. Add stevia to taste. Will keep, covered, in the refrigerator up to 5 days; may be frozen.

CHAPTER 12

Mains

Raw Sushi with Spicy Ginger-Miso Sauce
Good for: all stages

If you're missing sushi, don't despair. This raw recipe is filled with fresh veggies, including cauliflower, as a perfect stand-in for the rice (which is important especially if you're following the "Fast Track" version of the ACD and avoiding grains). The spicy sauce really brings these to the next level, so don't omit it.

MAKES 4 TO 6 SERVINGS

Spicy Ginger-Miso Sauce
2 teaspoons (10 ml) grated fresh ginger
2 teaspoons (10 ml) mellow miso
2 teaspoons (10 ml) tahini (sesame paste)
2 tablespoons (30 ml) Bragg Liquid Aminos or wheat-free tamari
Up to ⅛ teaspoon (0.5 ml) cayenne pepper, or to taste

"Rice"
1 small cauliflower, cut into florets (4 to 6 cups, or about 1 pound [500 g] florets)
2 tablespoons plus 2 teaspoons (40 ml) raw apple cider vinegar

4 teaspoons (20 ml) toasted sesame oil
5 drops plain pure liquid stevia, or to taste
Fine sea salt

For assembly
4 to 6 sheets nori
1 small carrot, peeled and cut into matchsticks
¼ cucumber, peeled and cut into matchsticks
½ sweet red bell pepper, cored and cut into matchsticks
½ small avocado, peeled, pitted, and cut into slices
Other add-ins, if desired: chopped fresh cilantro, shredded
    carrot, shredded daikon radish or jicama, thinly sliced
    fennel
Bragg Liquid Aminos, for dipping

Prepare the sauce: In a small bowl, mix all the ingredients together until smooth. It should be the consistency of a thick ketchup. If the mixture is too thick, add a bit of water and mix again until your desired consistency is reached.

Make the "rice": Using a food processor, pulse the cauliflower until it is broken up into small, ricelike pieces (take care not to overprocess, however, or you will have mush!). Add the remaining ingredients and pulse just until incorporated. Set aside.

Assemble the sushi: Place a sheet of nori, textured side up, on a cutting board or sushi mat. Spread a thin layer of the spicy miso sauce across the bottom edge, 1 to 2 inches wide. Spread about one quarter of the "rice" over the entire sheet, covering the sauce and leaving about 1 inch (2.5 cm) uncovered at the top edge of the sheet (opposite side from the sauce). Line up the carrot, cucumber, pepper, and avocado across the bottom edge, over where the sauce had been spread. Beginning at the side with the vegetables, tightly roll the nori sheet, jelly-roll style, stopping at the uncovered edge. Dip a finger in water and moisten across the uncovered edge of the nori, then continue to roll over that edge so that it is on the bottom of the roll (touching the mat). Using a sharp knife, cut across the roll to create bite-size pieces of sushi. Serve with Bragg Liquid Aminos and any extra sauce for dipping.

Super Stuffed Sweet Potatoes with Creamy Greens and Chickpeas
Good for: all stages

Baked sweet potatoes stuffed with greens and chickpeas is a perfect quick and nutrient-dense meal. The slightly sweet, soft sweet potato pairs well with a wide array of stuffings. Feel free to use other vegetable combinations on top of your spuds, too, to suit your tastes (and what's in your fridge); I also enjoy these topped with Beans Paprikash (page 191).

MAKES 2 MAIN COURSE SERVINGS

2 large sweet potatoes (about 12 ounces [350 g])
1 recipe Creamy Greens with Asian Seasonings (page 174)
1 large tomato, chopped, or about 1 cup [240 ml] chopped grape tomatoes
1½ cups (360 ml) cooked or canned chickpeas, rinsed and drained
⅓ cup (80 ml) raw or lightly toasted sunflower seeds
½ cup (120 ml) sunflower sprouts (optional)

Preheat the oven to 425°F (210°C). Bake the potatoes on a parchment-lined cookie sheet until soft, for 45 minutes to 1 hour.

About 20 minutes before the potatoes are ready, prepare the greens. To the pan of finished Creamy Greens, add the tomato and chickpeas and stir well. Lower the heat to low and keep warm until the potatoes are ready.

To serve, cut each sweet potato in half lengthwise. Top with about half of the greens mixture, then sprinkle with sunflower seeds and sprouts, if using. Serve.

Chickpea "Quiche"
Good for: all stages

This is a great brunch or light dinner meal-in-a-pan. The texture is somewhat like that of a crustless quiche, soft yet firm enough to hold its shape. The slices can be wrapped and saved for another day (they hold up well for packaged lunches, or even as a sandwich filling) or frozen for a quick meal down the road. The quiche also works nicely if made without the vegetables, then spread with either Sweet or Savory Almond Sauce (page 178) and topped with sliced apple or cranberries for a lovely brunch dish.

MAKES 6 TO 8 SERVINGS

Base
Coconut oil, for pan
2¼ cups (225 g) chickpea flour
2 tablespoons (30 ml) extra-virgin olive oil, preferably organic
¼ teaspoon (1 ml) fine sea salt, or to taste
3⅛ cups (750 ml) filtered water or vegetable broth or stock
   (use water for a sweet quiche)

Filling
½ bunch thin leafy greens, such as dandelion, chard, or spinach
   (about 4 cups/1 L chopped, unpacked), chopped or shredded
4 large garlic cloves, sliced
1 cup (240 ml) Oven-Dried Tomatoes (page 106)
½ cup (120 ml) cored and diced red or other sweet pepper or
   trimmed broccoli or zucchini

Preheat the oven to 475°F (245°C). Lightly grease a 9- or 10-inch (22.5 or 25 cm) cast-iron skillet or quiche pan with coconut oil and place in the preheated oven for 5 to 8 minutes. (Note: If you have a casserole dish that can withstand this kind of heat, you can use that instead.)

Prepare the base: Place the chickpea flour, oil, salt, and water in a large blender and blend until smooth and frothy. (Don't skip this step; it's essential to blend the flour to achieve the correct texture in the final dish.) Pour into a large bowl and mix in the prepared vegetables.

Once the skillet is heated, remove from the oven and pour the quiche batter into it. Using a silicone spatula, spread the veggies around so they are evenly distributed.

Bake for 15 to 18 minutes. Remove from the heat, rotate the pan, and return it to the oven for another 10 to 15 minutes, until somewhat puffed and browned on the edges. Remove from the heat and allow to cool for 10 minutes before slicing. May be frozen.

Pumpkin Patties
Good for: all stages

I love veggie burgers but find many of them don't hold their shape well when cooked; these patties stay together beautifully. They make a great light dinner with some homemade ketchup and a green salad, but their flavor is mild enough that they'd work great at a brunch table, too. And baking them results in firmer patties with a lovely, crisp exterior.

MAKES 8 TO 10 PATTIES

¼ cup (45 g) uncooked quinoa
1 small onion, coarsely chopped
⅔ cup (160 ml) pumpkin puree (or use butternut or acorn
      squash, but the patties will have a subtle sweetness in that
      case)
⅔ cup (65 g) chickpea flour
¼ cup (60 ml) coconut flour
1 tablespoon (15 ml) psyllium husks
1 tablespoon (15 ml) finely ground flaxseeds
¾ teaspoon (3.5 ml) baking powder
Fine sea salt
2 tablespoons (30 ml) extra-virgin olive oil, preferably organic
⅔ cup (160 ml) vegetable broth or stock
2 teaspoons (10 ml) raw apple cider vinegar
½ small jalapeño pepper, chopped (remove seeds for less heat)
1 tablespoon (15 ml) dried parsley, or 3 tablespoons (45 ml)
      chopped fresh

Preheat the oven to 350°F (180°C). Line a cookie sheet with parchment.

Grind the quinoa in a coffee grinder until powdered. Place in the bowl of a food processor along with all the other ingredients and process until almost smooth (you might want a bit of texture from the onion). Lift the blade and scrape under it, then pulse one or two more times to be sure everything is incorporated.

Using a large ice-cream scoop or a ⅓ cup (80 ml) measuring cup, scoop the "dough" onto the cookie sheet and flatten each slightly to form patties. Bake for 30 minutes, then flip the patties and continue to bake for another 15 minutes, or until browned. May be frozen.

Herbed Grain-Free Gnocchi
Good for: all stages

My favorite form of pasta before the ACD was gnocchi, so I was determined to re-create it in a form I could enjoy. Even without the wheat flour or starchy potatoes, this grain-free rendition of the classic really satisfies. These gnocchi are great topped with spicy tomato sauce or simply sautéed in some coconut oil and garlic.

SERVES 2 TO 4

¼ cup (60 ml) smooth natural almond butter or sunflower
   seed butter
⅔ cup (160 ml) vegetable broth or stock
¼ cup (60 ml) chopped fresh herbs of choice (I like basil,
   cilantro, parsley, and/or dill)
1¼ cups (125 g) chickpea flour, plus about ¼ cup (60 ml) for
   molding gnocchi
½ teaspoon (2.5 ml) baking powder
2 tablespoons (30 ml) whole psyllium husks
Pinch of fine sea salt, or to taste

In a medium-size bowl, whisk together the almond butter and broth. Add the herbs and stir to combine. Sift in the chickpea flour, baking powder, psyllium, and salt and stir well until you have a soft dough. Allow to rest for 2 to 5 minutes.

Sprinkle a cutting board with about ¼ cup (60 ml) of chickpea flour. Divide the dough into three roughly equal parts, and roll each to form a long rope about ½ inch (1.5 cm) thick. Cut the roll into pieces about 1 inch (2.5 cm) long. Dip a fork into more flour and press down on each piece to create light indentations.

To cook the gnocchi, bring a large pot of water to a boil, then lower the heat to medium-low. Using a large spoon, gently lower ten to twelve gnocchi at a time into the pot, and allow them to cook for 3 to 5 minutes (they will float to the top; cook for another 1 to 2 minutes after they do so). Use a slotted spoon to transfer the cooked gnocchi to a heatproof plate or bowl. You can keep them warm in a low temperature oven, about 275°F (135°C), while you repeat the process with the rest of the dough.

Serve with pasta sauce or sauté in some olive or coconut oil and garlic.

Pumpkin Dal
Good for: all stages

I'm wild about Indian food and love experimenting with all the spice mixtures that cuisine has to offer. This isn't a traditional dal (which doesn't usually feature pumpkin), but more like a fusion dish that's inspired by dal. Either way, it makes a delicious soup or stew, depending on how long you cook it and how thick you let the sauce become.

MAKES 6 TO 8 SERVINGS

2 tablespoons (30 ml) extra-virgin olive oil, preferably organic

1 large onion, chopped

3 garlic cloves, minced

1 large tomato, chopped

1 tablespoon (15 ml) minced fresh ginger

1 teaspoon (5 ml) ground cumin

½ teaspoon (5 ml) ground turmeric

1 teaspoon (5 ml) ground cinnamon

1½ teaspoons (7.5 ml) garam masala

½ teaspoon (5 ml) whole mustard seeds (I use yellow, but black would be fine)

1 bay leaf

½ small jalapeño pepper, chopped (remove seeds for less heat)

Fine sea salt

1 cup (240 ml) dried brown or green lentils, picked over to remove stones and washed

1 cup (240 ml) pure pumpkin or squash puree

3 cups (720 ml) vegetable broth or stock

3 drops plain pure liquid stevia (optional)

1 tablespoon (15 ml) freshly squeezed lemon juice

4 cups (1 L) loosely packed chopped dark leafy greens (e.g., chard, kale, collards, or baby spinach)

3 to 4 cups (720 to 960 ml) cooked brown rice, for serving (optional)

In a large pot or Dutch oven, heat the oil and add the onion and garlic. Sauté until the onion is translucent, for 5 to 7 minutes. Add the tomato, ginger, spices, bay leaf, and jalapeño and continue to cook for another 2 minutes. If the mixture begins to scorch, splash with about ¼ cup (60 ml) of the broth to deglaze the pan.

Add the remaining ingredients and bring to a boil; lower the heat to a simmer, cover the pot, and cook, stirring occasionally, until the lentils are soft and the liquid has cooked down and thickened to your desired thickness, for 50 to 75 minutes. Taste and adjust the salt, if necessary. Remove the bay leaf. Serve over brown rice, if desired. May be frozen.

Beans Paprikash
Good for: all stages

The combination of rich, creamy sauce with lots and lots of paprika, plus beans and greens makes for a delicious mix of flavors and textures. Pair with a side salad or hearty piece of Grain-Free Sandwich Bread (page 102) and you've got a robust, satisfying meal. This dish was one of the most popular recipes among the cookbook testers; I think you'll love it, too.

MAKES 4 SERVINGS

1 tablespoon (15 ml) extra-virgin olive oil, preferably organic
1 large onion, diced
2 garlic cloves, minced
1 tablespoon (15 ml) mild miso
1 cup (240 ml) canned full-fat coconut milk, preferably organic
1 cup (240 ml) vegetable broth or stock
2 cups (480 ml) cooked or canned white beans (white kidney
    beans are great in this), well drained and rinsed
1 tablespoon (15 ml) paprika
½ teaspoon (2.5 ml) fine sea salt, or to taste
Freshly ground black pepper
4 large chard or collard leaves, stems removed, shredded
¼ cup (60 ml) chopped fresh cilantro (optional)
1 tablespoon (15 ml) freshly squeezed lemon juice
2 cups (480 ml) cooked quinoa, buckwheat, or brown rice
    (from about ¾ cup [360 ml] dried])
1 medium-size avocado, peeled, pitted, and sliced (optional)

In a large skillet, heat the oil over medium heat. Add the onion and garlic and sauté until the onion is translucent, for 5 to 8 minutes.

In a small bowl, whisk together the miso and about 2 tablespoons (30 ml) of the coconut milk until smooth. Add this to the pot along with the rest of the coconut milk, and the broth, beans, paprika, salt, pepper, and chard. Break up the beans a bit with the back of a spoon, but leave most of them whole.

Cook, stirring frequently, until the mixture is thick and saucy and the chard is wilted, for 10 to 15 minutes. Add the cilantro, if using, and lemon juice, and cook for another 5 minutes.

Distribute the quinoa among four bowls and ladle the bean mixture on top. Serve with sliced avocado, if desired. May be frozen.

Eggplant "Parmesan"
Good for: all stages

When my sisters and I were growing up, my mom would bake eggplant parmesan at least once a month. We all loved the rich tomato sauce and gooey cheese. I decided I had to reproduce my own ACD-friendly version of the recipe that I could enjoy. This dish is so hearty, it will satisfy even the most staunch omnivore. My husband actually thought there was meat in this! It's a bit of work, but the tomato sauce can be made in advance and frozen until needed. The baked dish also freezes beautifully.

MAKES 6 SUBSTANTIAL SERVINGS

Eggplant
⅓ cup (50 g) coconut flour
½ cup (85 g) natural raw almonds
1 tablespoon (15 ml) chickpea flour
½ teaspoon (2.5 ml) sweet or smoked paprika
¼ teaspoon (1 ml) fine sea salt
½ cup (120 ml) vegetable broth or stock
1 medium-size eggplant, peeled and cut into ½-inch (1.3 cm)
    slices (about 10 slices)

Sauce
1 tablespoon (15 ml) extra-virgin olive oil, preferably organic
1 medium-size onion, chopped
4 garlic cloves, minced

½ medium-size green bell pepper, cored and diced (about 1 cup [240 ml])

2 celery stalks, diced

½ cup (120 ml) vegetable broth or stock

1 (28-ounce [796 ml]) can crushed tomatoes

5 drops plain pure liquid stevia (optional; this mellows the acid in the tomatoes)

1 tablespoon (15 ml) dried parsley, or ¼ cup (60 ml) chopped fresh

2 teaspoons (10 ml) dried oregano

1 tablespoon (15 ml) dried basil, or ¼ cup (60 ml) chopped fresh

Cheese

½ cup (80 g) raw cashews

3 tablespoons (45 ml) raw shelled hemp seeds (hemp hearts)

1 cup (240 ml) well-cooked white beans, well drained

Juice of ½ lemon (about 2 tablespoons [30 ml])

2 garlic cloves, sliced

½ medium-size red bell pepper, cored and cut into large chunks

½ teaspoon (2.5 ml) smoked paprika

1 tablespoon (15 ml) raw apple cider vinegar

½ teaspoon (2.5 ml) dry mustard

1 tablespoon (15 ml) chickpea or Garfava flour

2 teaspoons (10 ml) mellow miso (white or yellow)

⅓ cup (80 ml) vegetable broth or stock

⅔ cup (160 ml) unsweetened almond milk or coconut beverage (the kind in a carton)

Preheat the oven to 375°F (190°C). Line an 8 ½-inch (22 cm) square pan with parchment, or grease with coconut oil. Line two cookie sheets with parchment.

Bake the eggplant: In the bowl of a food processor, combine the coconut flour, almonds, chickpea flour, paprika, and salt and blend until the mixture has the consistency of bread crumbs. Transfer to a large bowl or deep plate. Place the broth in a bowl big enough to fit the largest slice of eggplant.

Dip each slice of eggplant in the broth, then coat with the crumbly mixture. Place the slices on the prepared cookie sheets as they are ready. Bake the eggplant for 30 to 40 minutes, until the slices are soft and the coating has begun to brown and crisp up. Remove from the oven and set aside until ready to use.

Make the sauce: While the eggplant bakes, heat the oil in a large pot over medium heat and add the onion, garlic, bell pepper, and celery. Sauté until the onion is translucent, for 8 to 10 minutes. Add the broth, cover the pot, and lower the heat. Simmer until the broth is completely absorbed, for 10 to 15 minutes. Add the remaining sauce ingredients, increase the heat to medium, and allow to come to a boil. If you have a splatter screen, this is a good time to use it. Lower the heat to a simmer and continue to cook the sauce, stirring occasionally, until the color darkens and the sauce is thick, for about 30 minutes.

Prepare the cheese: While the sauce simmers, combine all the cheese ingredients in a high-powered blender and blend until smooth. Transfer to a medium-size pot and cook over medium heat, stirring frequently, until the mixture bubbles and begins to darken, for about 5 minutes. Remove from the heat.

Assemble the dish: Spread a thin layer of the sauce (about one ladleful) over the bottom of the pan. Top with a single layer of eggplant slices, using about half of the slices to cover as much of the pan as you can. Spread about half of the remaining sauce over the eggplant, then pour about half of the cheese over the tomato sauce, gently spreading to coat. Top with the remaining eggplant, tomato sauce, and cheese. Bake until completely heated through, the top is dry, and the edges are bubbling, for 35 to 45 minutes. Allow to sit for 10 minutes before slicing.

May be frozen; place slices on a parchment-lined cookie sheet and freeze on the sheet until firm, then wrap each slice individually and freeze in a bag or container.

Veggie Fried Quinoa (or Rice) with Arame and Edamame
Good for: all stages

Seaweed is a great anticandida food (one you should try to incorporate as often as possible), and it works beautifully in this dish. This stir-fry is one of my favorite one-pot meals; between the vibrant colors of the veggies and the protein of the edamame, it's pretty and filling at the same time. Feel free to switch out some of the vegetables for others that you prefer; this is a very forgiving recipe!

MAKES 4 TO 6 SERVINGS

About ½ cup (120 ml) loosely packed dried arame (see tip)

1 cup (240 ml) warm filtered water

1 tablespoon (15 ml) virgin coconut or olive oil, preferably organic

1 large onion, chopped

4 garlic cloves, chopped

1 large carrot, sliced into rounds

1 cup (240 ml) cauliflower florets

1 cup (240 ml) broccoli florets

1 cup (240 ml) thinly sliced green or red cabbage

1 small zucchini, sliced lengthwise and then into half-moons

1 medium-size sweet red pepper, cored and diced

3 cups (720 ml) thinly sliced chard or collard leaves

1 cup (240 ml) shelled and cooked edamame

¼ to ½ cup (60 to 120 ml) water or vegetable broth or stock, if needed

2 cups (480 ml) cooked quinoa or brown basmati rice

3 tablespoons (45 ml) Bragg Liquid Aminos or wheat-free tamari, or to taste

2 teaspoons (10 ml) freshly squeezed lemon juice

2 tablespoons (30 ml) sesame seeds, for garnish (optional)

¼ cup (60 ml) chopped fresh cilantro leaves, for garnish (optional).

Place the arame in a small bowl and pour the warm water over it. Set aside.

Meanwhile, heat the oil in a large wok, skillet, or Dutch oven over medium heat. Add the onion and garlic and sauté until the onion is translucent, for 8 to 10 minutes. Add the carrot, cauliflower, broccoli, cabbage, and zucchini and continue to cook, stirring frequently, for another 5 minutes. Add the red pepper, chard, and edamame and stir to combine. If the mixture is very dry, add broth to prevent scorching. Cover and cook for about 5 minutes more, until the chard is wilted.

Drain the arame and add it to the pot along with the quinoa, liquid aminos, and lemon juice; stir until everything is well coated. Taste and add more liquid aminos if desired. Continue to cook until heated through. Serve with a sprinkling of sesame seeds and chopped cilantro, if desired. May be frozen.

Tip: Although it resembles black spaghetti when wet, dried arame (as it's sold) is light and somewhat fragile. When measuring, you want to set it lightly in the measuring cup, allowing the air spaces between threads to remain. Packing it will result in much more arame than you'll need! While it's not an exact science, handling your arame gently before soaking will prevent any huge discrepancies in the final amount.

Sunday Night Roast
Good for: all stages

Not intended to imitate the flavor of beef, this roast will nevertheless provide omnivores with a richly flavored, savory main course that really satisfies. Much like a meat loaf, the roast is full-bodied and moist and holds up well when sliced. Try serving it alongside vegetables and potatoes, topped with Perfect Golden Gravy (page 177). I presented this roast at a holiday dinner and even avowed omnivores gobbled it up.

MAKES 4 TO 6 SERVINGS

2 tablespoons (30 ml) extra-virgin olive oil, preferably organic,
    plus more for brushing

1 large onion, chopped

1 large carrot, grated

1 celery stalk, sliced

3 garlic cloves, sliced

1 small sweet potato (8 ounces [250 g] once trimmed and
    peeled), grated

1 medium-size tomato, cut into chunks

1 cup (240 ml) vegetable broth or stock, plus more if needed

1 tablespoon (15 ml) Bragg Liquid Aminos or wheat-free tamari

1½ teaspoons (7.5 ml) raw apple cider vinegar

1 tablespoon (15 ml) dried basil

1 teaspoon (5 ml) dried oregano

¼ cup (60 ml) chopped fresh parsley

¼ cup (60 ml) chopped fresh cilantro (or use more parsley)

½ teaspoon (2.5 ml) smoked paprika

Fine sea salt (may not be necessary if your broth is salted)

⅓ cup (55 g) raw pumpkin seeds

½ cup (60 g) uncooked quinoa, ground into a powder in a
    coffee grinder

¾ cup (75 g) chickpea flour

½ teaspoon (2.5 ml) baking powder

Preheat the oven to 325°F (170°C). Line a cookie sheet with parchment.

In a large skillet, heat the oil and add the onion, carrot, celery, garlic, and sweet potato. Cook until the onion is translucent, for about 10 minutes. Add the tomato, broth, liquid aminos, vinegar, basil, oregano, parsley, cilantro, paprika, and salt; lower the heat to medium-low, cover, and cook until the sweet potato is soft and the broth is absorbed, for about 20 minutes (if the potato isn't quite ready by the time the liquid is absorbed, add up to ¼ cup [60 ml] more broth and keep cooking).

Meanwhile, in the bowl of a food processor, process the pumpkin seeds, quinoa powder, chick-pea flour, and baking powder until the mixture has the consistency of fine bread crumbs. Add the vegetable mixture to the processor and blend until well combined and a very soft dough (almost like a muffin batter) has formed. Allow to sit for 5 minutes.

Once the dough has rested for 5 minutes, turn the dough onto the prepared cookie sheet and, using a silicone spatula, shape it into an 8 x 5 x 3½-inch (20 x 12.5 x 9 cm) "roast" shape. Use the spatula to smooth the outside and create a domed top.

Bake for 50 to 55 minutes, until the top is dry and the edges are browned. Remove from the oven and brush with oil, then bake for an additional 15 to 25 minutes, or until the top is lightly browned.

Allow to cool completely before wrapping and refrigerating overnight. When ready to serve, cover with foil and reheat at 350°F (180°C) for about 25 minutes. Slice and serve. May be frozen.

Tempeh "Bourguignon"
Good for: all stages

Years ago, I spent a weekend visiting with one of my university mentors and his wife. She served boeuf bourguignon, a rich, slow-cooked stew, and I fell in love with the robust flavors. I remembered that magical weekend and the wonderful stew when I created this recipe. The secret ingredient that reproduces the savory umami of red wine in this bourguignon is unsweetened cranberry juice!

MAKES 4 SERVINGS

2 (.75-pound [350 g]) packages tempeh
3 tablespoons (45 ml) extra-virgin olive oil
2 tablespoons (30 ml) Bragg Liquid Aminos
2 medium-size onions, chopped
1 large leek, white and light green parts only, chopped
2 carrots, chopped
3 garlic cloves, minced

1 tablespoon (15 ml) dried parsley

1 tablespoon (15 ml) dried chives

½ teaspoon (2.5 ml) dried thyme

¼ teaspoon (1 ml) dried marjoram

2 bay leaves

½ teaspoon (2.5 ml) celery seeds

⅛ teaspoon (0.5 ml) ground cloves

Freshly ground black pepper

¼ teaspoon (1 ml) salt, or more to taste

1 cup (240 ml) vegetable broth or stock (preferably homemade)

½ cup (120 ml) unsweetened cranberry juice

5 to 10 drops plain pure liquid stevia

1 tablespoon (15 ml) tapioca or arrowroot starch (optional; omit for Stage 1)

Cooked rice or mashed potatoes, for serving

Cut the tempeh into bite-size pieces. Mix 1 tablespoon (15 ml) of the olive oil and the liquid aminos in the bottom of an ovenproof glass or ceramic square pan, and toss the tempeh to coat it evenly. Allow to marinate for at least 30 minutes.

Preheat the oven to 350°F (180°C). Bake the tempeh until the marinade is absorbed and the pieces are beginning to brown, for 15 to 20 minutes. Remove from the oven and allow to cool while you prepare the base.

In a large pot or Dutch oven, heat the remaining 2 tablespoons (30 ml) of olive oil over medium heat and add the onions, leek, and carrots. Sauté until the vegetables are softened but not browned, for 5 to 7 minutes. Add the garlic, parsley, and chives and cook for another 2 minutes. Add the remaining ingredients, except the tempeh and tapioca, and bring to a boil over medium heat. Add the tempeh, then lower the heat, cover, and simmer for 25 to 30 minutes, until much of the liquid is evaporated and the vegetables are beginning to dissolve into the sauce. If necessary, add the tapioca starch by mixing it in a small bowl with 2 to 3 tablespoons (30 to 45 ml) of the sauce first, then returning the mixture to the pot and stirring well. Remove the bay leaves.

To serve, spoon over cooked rice or mashed potatoes. May be frozen.

Zucchini Linguine with Lentil-Tomato Sauce
Good for: all stages

Zucchini strips stand in for the typical starchy noodles in this recipe, which is a great way to enjoy the experience of eating pasta without actually eating pasta. The sauce is surprisingly robust, as the rutabaga adds a savory, earthy quality without overpowering the flavors here. For another option, try the Herbed Grain-Free Gnocchi (page 188) instead of zucchini with this sauce.

MAKES 6 SERVINGS

1 tablespoon (15 ml) extra-virgin olive oil, preferably organic
1 large onion, finely chopped
4 garlic cloves, chopped
½ cup (120 ml) finely grated rutabaga
1 cup (240 ml) dried green lentils, rinsed and picked over
¼ cup (60 ml) dried red lentils
3½ to 4 cups (840 ml to 1 L) vegetable broth or stock, plus
    more if needed
1 (28-ounce [796 ml]) can crushed tomatoes
1 teaspoon (5 ml) dried oregano
1 tablespoon (15 ml) dried basil, or ¼ cup (60 ml), finely
    chopped fresh
¼ cup (60 ml) chopped fresh parsley
¼ teaspoon (1 ml) cayenne pepper, or ½ jalapeño pepper,
    minced (remove seeds for less heat)
Fine sea salt and freshly ground black pepper
3 medium-size zucchini, washed and ends trimmed

In a large pot, heat the olive oil over medium heat. Add the onion, garlic, and rutabaga. Lower the heat and sauté, stirring frequently, until the onion is golden, for about 7 minutes. Stir in the lentils along with the broth and bring to a boil.

Lower the heat and add the tomatoes, herbs, spices, and salt and pepper to taste. Cover and simmer, stirring occasionally, until the lentils are tender, for about 25 minutes. If the sauce begins to get too thick, add more stock, ¼ cup (60 ml) at a time, as needed.

Meanwhile, using a vegetable peeler, peel the zucchini lengthwise to create long strips, like linguine (alternatively, use a vegetable spiralizer to create the "pasta"). Place about 1 cup (240 ml) of the zucchini on each plate and top with the sauce. Serve immediately. The sauce may be frozen.

Grain and Veggie Meal-in-a-Bowl
Good for: all stages

I'm a huge fan of meals-in-a-bowl. Typically, such bowls contain a mix of salad greens and/or cooked veggies, a grain, one or two forms of protein (e.g., tempeh, nuts, seeds, or legumes) and a flavorful sauce to bring it all together. Once you've tried this recipe, you'll find it easy to come up with your own new combinations, too.

MAKES 4 SERVINGS

2½ cups (600 ml) vegetable broth or stock, plus more if
    needed
1 cup (240 ml) uncooked millet, quinoa, or buckwheat
1 small eggplant, cut into ½-inch (1.3 cm) slices
1 medium-size zucchini, cut into 1-inch (2.5 cm) slices
1 medium-size sweet red bell pepper, cut into chunks
Olive oil
2 teaspoons (10 ml) dried oregano (optional)
2 teaspoons (10 ml) dried basil (optional)
½ teaspoon (2.5 ml) fine sea salt, or to taste
4 cups (1 L) mixed baby greens, baby kale, or baby spinach
1 recipe Sweet or Savory Almond Sauce, page 178; Garlicky
    Warm Avocado Sauce, page 179; Fresh Spicy Tomato
    Dressing or Sauce, page 180; or any of the other dressings
    in the book
4 green onions, sliced
½ cup (120 ml) raw or lightly toasted sunflower seeds
1 avocado, peeled, pitted, and sliced

Preheat the oven to 425°F (220°C). Line a cookie sheet with parchment.

In a medium-size pot over high heat, bring the broth to a boil. Add the millet, lower the heat to low, cover the pot, and allow the millet to cook undisturbed for 20 minutes. After 20 minutes, check to see whether all the water is absorbed. If it's not, cover and continue to cook until the grains are dry and all the liquid is gone. If it's too dry, add up to ¼ cup (60 ml) more liquid, and continue to cook until the grains are done. Set aside.

Meanwhile, roast the vegetables: Place the chopped vegetables in a bowl, drizzle with oil, and sprinkle with the oregano and basil, if using, and salt; toss until the veggies are well coated. Transfer the vegetables to the prepared cookie sheet and spread out in a single layer. Bake for 20 to 25 minutes, until the vegetables are just tender and slightly browned in places.

Assemble the bowl: Place about 1 cup (120 ml) of greens in the bottom of the bowl, and top with about ¾ cup (180 ml) of the cooked grains. Top with about one quarter of the grilled vegetables. Drizzle with your choice of sauce, then sprinkle with green onion and sunflower seeds. Place a few slices of avocado on the side and serve.

Creamy Black Beans and Rutabaga Stew with Baharat Blend
Good for: all stages

This stew is seasoned with my homemade version of African Baharat blend, a fragrant and alluring combination of sweet and hot spices, such as cinnamon, cumin, chili, and cloves. When mixed together, the sum of the parts is truly irresistible; I found myself returning to the kitchen over and over while the stew simmered, drawn by the magnetic aroma of this enticing sauce.

MAKES 6 TO 8 SERVINGS

Stew

2 tablespoons (30 ml) extra-virgin olive oil, preferably organic

1 large onion, chopped

2 cups (480 ml) diced rutabaga, cut into ½-inch (1.3 cm) dice (be sure the pieces are not too big or they won't cook properly!)

3 garlic cloves, minced

1 cup (240 ml) vegetable broth or stock

¾ cup (180 ml) seeded and diced red bell pepper

A small bunch of chard or lacinato kale leaves (5 to 7 medium-size leaves), stems removed, shredded

1½ to 2 cups (360 to 480 ml) well-cooked, drained black beans (canned is fine)

Sauce

½ cup (120 ml) smooth natural almond butter

1 teaspoon (5 ml) ground coriander

1 teaspoon (5 ml) ground cinnamon

¼ teaspoon (1 ml) ground cloves or allspice

½ teaspoon (2.5 ml) ground cumin

⅛ teaspoon (0.5 ml) ground cardamom

¼ teaspoon (1 ml) ground nutmeg

2 teaspoons (10 ml) sweet or smoked paprika

1 teaspoon (5 ml) mild curry powder

½ to ¾ cup (120 to 180 ml) vegetable broth or stock

1 tablespoon (15 ml) freshly squeezed lemon juice

5 drops plain pure liquid stevia, or to taste

Fine sea salt

Chopped fresh cilantro, for garnish

Cooked brown rice or quinoa for serving, if desired

Cook the vegetables: In a large pot or nonstick skillet, heat the oil over medium heat and add the onion and rutabaga. Cook until the onion is translucent and the rutabaga begins to darken, for 8 to 10 minutes. Add the garlic and cook for another 2 minutes. Add the broth and cook, covered, until all the liquid is absorbed and the rutabaga is soft, for 15 to 20 minutes, stirring occasionally.

Meanwhile, make the sauce: Combine all the ingredients except the lemon juice, stevia, salt, cilantro, and brown rice in a bowl or glass measuring cup and whisk until smooth.

Once the rutabaga is cooked, add the red pepper, chard, beans, and sauce and stir gently to combine and coat everything in sauce. Lower the heat, then cover and continue to cook gently until everything is warmed through and the greens are wilted, for 5 to 10 minutes. Stir in the lemon juice and stevia and adjust the seasonings, then garnish with cilantro and serve (either as is or over rice or quinoa).

CHAPTER 13

Sweets

Homemade Chocolate
Good for: all stages (see note)

This recipe is very versatile—you can use it for chocolate chips or bars, and it's great with add-ins for a sweet treat when you're missing chocolate. Be sure to use raw cacao, though, as regular cocoa is too bitter for this recipe.

MAKES 3 TO 4 SERVINGS

- 1 tablespoon (15 ml) cacao butter (you can grate it and then melt it to measure)
- 1 tablespoon (15 ml) coconut oil
- 2 teaspoons (10 ml) smooth natural cashew butter
- 1 tablespoon (15 ml) raw cacao powder
- 1 tablespoon (15 ml) carob powder
- 1 teaspoon (5 ml) raw vanilla powder, or ½ teaspoon (2.5 ml) pure vanilla extract
- 15 to 20 drops (or more, to taste) vanilla, chocolate, or hazelnut-flavored pure liquid stevia
- Pinch of fine sea salt
- Optional add-ins: up to 2 tablespoons (30 ml) total, any combination of cacao nibs, chopped nuts or seeds, and/or coconut or allowed dried fruits

In a small pot or bowl set over simmering water, melt the cacao butter, coconut oil, and cashew butter together. Whisk in the remaining ingredients until smooth. Pour into a small square container lined with plastic wrap (to make chips), small silicone molds, or ice cube trays, or use melted as a dip for truffles.

Refrigerate until firm, for at least 1 hour. For chips, turn the chocolate out of the mold and onto a cutting board. Using a very sharp knife, cut into small chunks. Store in an airtight container in the fridge for up to 2 weeks. May be frozen. Not suitable for baking, unfortunately (they won't hold their shape if baked), but great in ice cream or truffles. (For chips you can use in baking, replace the coconut oil with another 1 tablespoon (15 ml) of cacao butter).

Note: If you find that raw cacao triggers cravings for you, you may not be able to enjoy this chocolate in Stage 1 of the diet. You can use carob powder instead of the cacao here for a caffeine-free and still very tasty treat (in that case, add another teaspoon (5 ml) of coconut oil to the mixture).

Grain-Free Fudgy Brownies or Fudgy Brownie Cookies
Good for: all stages (see note)

Yes, Virginia, there is a fudgy brownie recipe on an anticandida diet! Filled with high-fiber, low-glycemic ingredients, this brownie is nevertheless fudgy, chocolaty, and delicious.

MAKES 9 TO 12 SQUARES OR 12 TO 15 COOKIES

½ cup (120 ml) sweet potato puree
¼ cup (60 ml) yacon syrup
¼ cup (60 ml) smooth natural almond butter or tahini (sesame paste)
2 tablespoons (30 ml) tahini (sesame seed paste)
3 tablespoons (45 ml) coconut oil, preferably organic, at room temperature
1 tablespoon (15 ml) finely ground flaxseeds
1 tablespoon (15 ml) pure vanilla extract

½ teaspoon (2.5 ml) pure almond extract (optional)

20 to 40 drops plain, vanilla, or chocolate-flavored pure liquid
   stevia

⅓ cup (80 ml) chopped nuts or seeds, or homemade carob
   chips (see Homemade Chocolate, page 205)

3 tablespoons (45 ml) raw or toasted whole buckwheat groats
   or whole quinoa (see note)

½ cup (60 g) raw cacao powder (see note)

½ teaspoon (2.5 ml) baking powder

¼ teaspoon (1 ml) baking soda

¾ teaspoon (3.5 ml) xanthan gum

¼ teaspoon (1 ml) fine sea salt

Preheat the oven to 350°F (180°C). Line an 8-inch (20 cm) square pan, or an 8-inch (20 cm) loaf pan and one cookie sheet, or two cookie sheets with parchment.

In a medium-size bowl or food processor, blend together the sweet potato puree, yacon syrup, almond butter, tahini, coconut oil, flaxseeds, vanilla, almond extract, if using, and stevia. If mixing by hand, whisk well to ensure everything is smooth and well blended. Stir in the nuts. Set aside.

In a coffee or spice grinder, grind the buckwheat to a fine powder. Sift into a medium-size bowl with the carob powder, baking powder, baking soda, xanthan gum, and salt. Whisk to combine. Pour the wet mixture over the dry and stir well. You should end up with a very thick batter or soft dough, like a cookie dough. Resist the urge to add more liquid!

Turn the mixture into the prepared square pan; or turn half into the loaf pan and leave half in the bowl for cookies. Spread and flatten with a rubber or silicone spatula or the palms of your hands (it should be too thick to pour; you will have to spread it out, like a dough). For cookies, scoop onto the prepared cookie sheet, using a small ice-cream scoop or teaspoon, and then flatten the mounds to about ¼ inch (6 mm) thick (the cookies won't spread much).

Bake for 15 to 20 minutes for the square pan, for 12 to 15 minutes for the loaf pan, and 8 to 9 minutes for the cookies, rotating the pans about halfway through. The mixture should look dry on top but be very soft to the touch, and a knife inserted in the center will come out clean. Do not overbake.

Allow to cool completely in the pan, then refrigerate until cold before slicing (they will tend to fall apart otherwise). For cookies, allow to cool for 5 minutes on the pans, then transfer to a wire rack to cool completely. Store in an airtight container in the fridge for up to 4 days, or freeze.

Note: If you use toasted buckwheat, you will taste buckwheat flavor in your brownie. I happen to like the flavor, but, if you're not a fan, aim for raw buckwheat groats or quinoa instead.

Note: If you find that raw cacao triggers cravings for you, you may not be able to use it in Stage 1 of the diet. You can use carob powder instead of the cacao here for a tasty carob brownie instead (in that case, add another 2 tablespoons (30 ml) of coconut oil to the batter).

Q&E

Emergency Fudge
Good for: all stages

We've all been there: a serious, severe sweets craving. Fortunately, this quick and easy recipe satisfies without refined sugar. I've left this at a small batch so you don't have to worry if you happen to eat the entire thing (hypothetically, of course).

MAKES 2 SMALL OR 1 LARGE SERVING

1 tablespoon (15 ml) tahini (sesame paste)
1 tablespoon (15 ml) smooth natural almond butter or seed
    butter
2 teaspoons (10 ml) Homemade Coconut Butter (page 100)
10 to 15 drops plain or vanilla pure liquid stevia, or to taste
1 tablespoon (15 ml) carob powder

In a small bowl, mix all the ingredients well. Scoop onto a piece of plastic wrap and shape into a small log or bar. Chill in the refrigerator for at least 30 minutes, or in the freezer for 3 to 5 minutes, until firm. Cut into small squares. If it's a true sweets emergency, just eat right away, using a spoon.

Raw Chocolate Chip Cookie Dough Truffles
Good for: all stages

Q&E

If you like raw cookie dough, you'll love these truffles. The texture and flavor of cookie dough, combined with a high-protein "secret ingredient," means this sweet snack provides a hefty nutritional punch, too! The recipe offers two variations: plain cookie dough balls or, for a richer treat, truffles dipped in chocolate. Either way, you will love them!

MAKES ABOUT 30 TRUFFLES (RECIPE MAY BE HALVED)

Truffles

1 cup (240 ml) well-cooked and drained chickpeas or white beans

2 tablespoons (30 ml) coconut sugar (see note)

3 tablespoons (45 ml) smooth natural seed or nut butter (I use almond butter)

1 tablespoon (15 ml) coconut oil

1 teaspoon (5 ml) ground cinnamon

2 teaspoons (10 ml) pure vanilla extract, or 2 teaspoons (10 ml) vanilla powder

⅛ teaspoon (0.5 ml) pure stevia powder, or ¼ teaspoon (1 ml) vanilla or chocolate-flavored pure liquid stevia, or to taste

3 tablespoons (45 ml) coconut flour

2½ tablespoons (37.5 ml) unflavored or vanilla raw protein powder (pea or rice)

Pinch of fine sea salt

3 tablespoons (45 ml) plain or vanilla unsweetened almond milk or other allowed nondairy milk or more, as needed

⅓ cup (80 ml) homemade carob or chocolate chips (page 205) or cacao nibs

Chocolate Coating (optional; makes enough for about 15 truffles)

¼ cup (30 g) raw cacao powder

3 tablespoons (45 ml) coconut oil

⅛ to ¼ teaspoon (0.5 to 1 ml) pure stevia powder, or ¼ to ½ teaspoon (1 to 2.5 ml) pure liquid stevia

½ teaspoon (2.5 ml) vanilla powder, or 1 teaspoon (5 ml) pure vanilla extract

Make the truffles: In the bowl of a food processor, process the chickpeas, coconut sugar, seed butter, coconut oil, cinnamon, vanilla, and stevia until very smooth. Add the coconut flour, protein powder, salt, and milk and process until the mixture comes together in a very soft dough. Stir in the chips by hand; don't process again.

As a snack, you can eat the dough right away.

For truffles, scoop about 1 tablespoon (15 ml) of the dough at a time and place on a cookie sheet. Freeze until just firm, then roll into balls. For uncoated truffles, store in a covered container in the refrigerator for up to 4 days, or freeze. If coating in chocolate, return the truffles to the freezer while you prepare the chocolate coating.

Make the coating: Place a medium-size metal or heatproof glass bowl over a small pot containing about 1 inch (2.5 cm) of simmering water (be sure that the bowl is big enough to cover the pot, and that it isn't actually touching the water). Place the coating ingredients in the bowl and stir frequently until everything is melted and smooth. Remove the bowl from the pot and turn off the heat.

To coat the truffles: Place a ball on a fork and dip into the chocolate, allowing any excess chocolate to drip back into the bowl. Tap the fork against the top of the bowl so that excess chocolate drips through the tines and back into the bowl. Slide the ball off the fork and back onto the cookie sheet, and repeat to coat the remaining balls. Return the cookie sheet to the freezer to chill just until firmed up. You may repeat the dipping process for a thicker chocolate coating. Store in a closed container in the refrigerator for up to 5 days. May be frozen.

Note: For Stage 1, omit the coconut sugar and use more stevia, to taste.

Raw Frosted "Put the Lime in the Coconut" Bars
Good for: all stages

A great no-bake dessert for warmer weather. With lime, ginger, and coconut, these delicious bars will bring a little of the tropics into your home.

MAKES 18 TO 20 BARS

Base
2 tablespoons (30 ml) finely ground chia seeds, preferably white seeds (from about 1 tablespoon [15 ml] whole seeds)

½ cup (75 g) raw or lightly toasted hazelnuts

½ cup (70 g) raw or lightly toasted pumpkin seeds

Pinch of fine sea salt

⅔ cup (70 g) unsweetened shredded coconut (use weight, as volume will differ depending on whether it's fine or medium shred)

Grated zest of 2 limes

2 teaspoons (10 ml) grated fresh ginger

Juice of 1 lime (about 2 tablespoons [30 ml])

40 drops plain or vanilla pure liquid stevia, or ¼ cup (60 ml) yacon syrup plus 20 drops pure liquid stevia

1 teaspoon (5 ml) pure vanilla extract

2 to 3 tablespoons (30 to 45 ml) water, if necessary

Frosting
2 tablespoons (30 ml) Homemade Coconut Butter (page 100), melted

2 tablespoons (30 ml) coconut oil

2 tablespoons (30 ml) smooth natural macadamia or cashew butter

Zest of 1 lime

Juice of 1 lime (about 2 tablespoons [30 ml])

Tiny pinch of fine sea salt

15 to 20 drops plain or vanilla pure liquid stevia, or more to taste

Make the base: Line a an 8-inch (20 cm) loaf pan with parchment or plastic wrap and set aside.

In the bowl of a food processor, process the chia seeds, hazelnuts, pumpkin seeds, and salt until the mixture resembles fine bread crumbs. Add the coconut, lime zest, and ginger and pulse to combine. In a small bowl, mix together the lime juice, stevia, and vanilla. Pour in a ring over the mixture in the processor bowl, then process until you have slightly moist dough that holds together when pinched between thumb and fingers. If the mixture is too dry, add the water and pulse to combine.

Press the base firmly into the prepared loaf pan and place in the refrigerator while you prepare the frosting.

Make the frosting: In a small food processor or blender, blend all the ingredients until smooth (the mixture may seem liquid at this point; this is fine). If the oil separates out, causing the mixture to appear curdled and too thick, add water, 1 tablespoon (15 ml) at a time, and blend again to emulsify. The frosting can be quite thin at this point (like a cake batter) but will firm up considerably in the refrigerator. Spread or pour the frosting over the base in the pan. Refrigerate until firm, for 2 to 4 hours. Remove from the pan and slice into small squares. May be frozen.

Vanilla Frosting: Omit the lime zest and juice; add 2 teaspoons (10 ml) of pure vanilla extract, and use 2 to 3 tablespoons (30 to 45 ml) of almond or coconut milk in place of the lime juice. Vanilla frosting also works well over Grain-Free Fudgy Brownies (page 206).

Grain-Free Apple Berry Crumble
Good for: Stage 2 and beyond

This fresh, not-too-sweet dessert is a great way to enjoy fruit once you reintroduce it to your diet. Because the topping is grain-free, you won't need to worry about consuming your coveted grain servings for dessert. For a real treat, top it with some Vanilla Ice Cream (page 220), or serve with Classic Whipped Cream (page 221).

MAKES 4 OR 6 SERVINGS

Filling

Coconut oil, for pan

2 small or 1 large sweet apple (I used Gala) or pear, cored and
diced very small (about ½-inch [1.3 cm] cubes—feel free
to leave the skin on)

1½ cups (360 ml) mixed fresh or frozen berries (not including
cranberries)—I use strawberries, raspberries, blackberries,
and blueberries; if cranberries are included in your mix, use
2 cups (480 ml) total

½ cup (120 ml) fresh or frozen cranberries

Zest of 1 lemon

1 teaspoon (5 ml) ground cinnamon

2 tablespoons (30 ml) freshly squeezed lemon juice (about ½
lemon)

¼ cup (60 ml) water

30 drops plain or fruit-flavored pure liquid stevia (I use 20
drops lemon and 10 drops cherry-vanilla)

1 teaspoon (5 ml) psyllium husks (optional—it prevents the
juices from becoming too watery)

Topping

⅓ cup (55 g) raw natural almonds

⅓ cup (55 g) raw sunflower or pumpkin seeds

2 tablespoons (30 ml) coconut flour

1/16 teaspoon (0.25 ml) pure stevia powder, or ⅛ teaspoon
(0.5 ml) pure liquid stevia, or to taste

1 tablespoon (15 ml) ground cinnamon

½ teaspoon (2.5 ml) ground ginger

⅛ teaspoon (0.5 ml) fine sea salt

1 tablespoon (15 ml) virgin coconut oil, preferably organic

Preheat the oven to 350°F (180°C). Grease a 4- to 6-cup (1 to 1.5 L) casserole dish with coconut oil.

Prepare the filling: In a large bowl, toss the apples, berries, cranberries, lemon zest, and cinnamon. In a small bowl, mix together the lemon juice, water, stevia, and psyllium, then drizzle over the berry mixture and toss again to coat evenly. Pour the mixture into the prepared casserole dish. (Note: You can just toss everything in the casserole dish instead of dirtying a bowl, but I found the mixture very hard to coat evenly when the ingredients were so cramped in the dish!)

Make the topping: In the bowl of a food processor, blend the almonds, seeds, coconut flour, stevia, cinnamon, ginger, and salt until the mixture resembles fine bread crumbs. Add the coconut oil and process until it's incorporated.

Sprinkle the topping evenly over the filling in the casserole dish. Bake for 35 to 45 minutes, rotating the dish about halfway through baking, until the topping is lightly browned and the filling is bubbly. Allow to cool somewhat before serving. May be frozen.

Avocado Mousse
Good for: all stages

Believe it or not, avocado can be a wonderful dessert ingredient, too. Here's a quick and easy mousse that can be eaten on its own with a sprinkling of nuts or seeds, or used as a topper for pancakes, waffles, or berries. However you enjoy it, it's irresistible.

MAKES 4 SERVINGS

1 (14-ounce [400 ml]) can full-fat coconut milk
1 small or medium-size barely ripe avocado (use a small one
    for milder flavor—but be sure it isn't overly ripe!), pitted
    and scooped from peel
20 to 30 drops plain or vanilla pure liquid stevia, or to your
    taste

1 teaspoon (5 ml) pure vanilla extract, or 1 teaspoon (5 ml)
    pure vanilla powder
1 teaspoon (5 ml) freshly squeezed lemon juice
½ teaspoon (2.5 ml) almond extract (optional)
¼ teaspoon (1 ml) xanthan gum (optional)

In a high-speed blender or food processor, blend all the ingredients, except the xanthan gum, until perfectly smooth. Add the xanthan and stir by hand just to incorporate, then blend until well combined and thickened. Transfer to a covered container and refrigerate for at least 4 hours or up to overnight before using. Will keep, covered, in the refrigerator for up to 2 days.

Note: If you omit the xanthan gum, the mousse will be denser and more like a pudding, but still delicious.

Crimson Mousse
Good for: all stages

Going without fruit on the first stage of the diet can be tough for some people. When I was yearning for a fruity sweet treat, I came up with this mousse recipe. Boiling the beets helps remove any trace of earthy flavor here; what remains is a vague sweetness and stunning hue. I served this dessert to friends at a dinner party and everyone guessed "berries" as the secret ingredient, even though they couldn't quite place them!

MAKES 4 SERVINGS

1 medium-size beet, peeled and diced very small (about 2
    ounces [55 g])
⅓ cup (55 g) raw cashews
1 cup (240 ml) canned full-fat coconut milk
2 tablespoons (30 ml) whole chia seeds, measured first and
    then ground in a coffee grinder to a fine powder
¼ teaspoon (1 ml) pure almond extract
¼ teaspoon (1 ml) coconut extract (optional)
1 teaspoon (5 ml) pure vanilla extract
15 to 25 drops plain or fruit-flavored pure liquid stevia, or to
    taste (I like cherry-vanilla)
1 tablespoon (15 ml) freshly squeezed lime juice
Pinch of fine sea salt
Classic Whipped Cream (page 221) (optional)

Place the beet in a small pot of water and bring to a boil. Cook for at least 30 minutes, until the beet is very soft and the water is deep crimson, and up to 50 minutes (the longer you cook them, the less they will retain their "beety" flavor). Drain well (reserve the liquid for soup or other uses).

Place the drained beet and the cashews, coconut milk, chia, almond extract, coconut extract, if using, vanilla, stevia, lime juice, and salt in a high-speed blender and blend until perfectly smooth, pushing the mousse down into the blades occasionally as necessary. Turn the mixture into a bowl, cover, and refrigerate for at least 4 hours or overnight (refrigerating allows the cashews to absorb some of the liquid and the mousse to thicken). Spoon or pipe into serving dishes and top with Classic Whipped Cream, if desired. Will keep, covered, in the refrigerator for up to 3 days.

If using a regular blender, blend the cashews, coconut milk, almond extract, coconut extract, if using, vanilla, stevia, lime juice, and salt until very smooth. Add the beets and blend again until smooth, then add the chia seeds last and blend just to combine. Pour into a bowl and refrigerate as directed.

Note: I've tried baking the beets instead of boiling, and while the color becomes even more intense in that case, so does the "beety" flavor; I wouldn't advise it.

Carob or Chocolate Pudding
Good for: all stages

You won't believe how rich and decadent this pudding tastes without dairy or sugar! Blended together, sweet potato and carob (or cacao) are truly a match made in culinary heaven.

MAKES 2 SERVINGS

½ cup (120 ml) baked sweet potato puree (about ½ sweet potato

½ cup (120 ml) canned coconut milk

3 tablespoons (45 ml) carob powder or raw cacao powder (see note)

¼ to ½ teaspoon (1 to 2.5 ml) pure liquid stevia (orange or vanilla works well)

Fine sea salt

⅓ cup (80 ml) Homemade Coconut Milk (page 99), or ¼ cup unsweetened almond milk

1 teaspoon (5 ml) ground cinnamon

Blend all the ingredients in a blender until smooth. For thicker pudding, refrigerate for 4 hours or overnight. Will keep, covered in the refrigerator, for up to 3 days.

Note: If you find that raw cacao triggers cravings for you, use the carob option here in Stage 1.

S'Mores Parfaits
Good for: all stages

With a grahamlike bottom layer, a fluffy marshmallow-like mousse filling and chocolate drizzle, these treats—often relegated to kids' campfires—are truly impressive, and delicious enough to serve to guests. (Note: You may use about ½ cup (120 ml) of homemade chocolate chips instead of the drizzle.)

MAKES 4 LARGE PARFAITS

Marshmallow Fluff

1 cup (160 g) raw cashews (see note)

⅔ cup (160 ml) canned full-fat coconut milk

⅔ cup filtered water or Homemade Coconut Milk (page 99)

2 teaspoons (10 ml) vanilla powder, or 1 tablespoon (15 ml)
    pure vanilla extract

¼ cup (40 g) whole chia seeds (use the white ones if you can
    find them)

Pinch of fine sea salt

¹⁄₁₆ to ⅛ teaspoon (0.25 to 0.5 ml) stevia powder or pure liquid
    stevia

"Graham Cracker" Crumble

½ cup (55 g) raw walnut pieces or halves

¼ cup (40 g) raw shelled hemp seeds (hemp hearts)

4 teaspoons (20 ml) lucuma (or carob powder for Stage 1)

⅛ teaspoon (0.5 ml) fine sea salt

2½ tablespoons (37.5 ml) coconut flour

⅛ to ¼ teaspoon (0.5 to 1 ml) pure stevia powder, or ¼ to ½
    teaspoon (1 to 2.5 ml) pure liquid stevia, or to taste

1 teaspoon (5 ml) ground cinnamon

2 teaspoons (10 ml) pure vanilla extract

2 tablespoons (30 ml) unsweetened almond or other nondairy
    milk of choice

Chocolate Drizzle

¼ cup (30 g) raw cacao powder (see note)

3 tablespoons (45 ml) coconut oil

⅛ to ¼ teaspoon (0.5 to 1 ml) pure stevia powder, or ¼ to ½
    teaspoon (1 to 2.5 ml) liquid stevia

½ teaspoon (2.5 ml) vanilla powder, or 1 teaspoon (5 ml) pure
    vanilla extract

Make the fluff: In a high-powered blender, combine all the ingredients and blend, using the tamper to push the ingredients toward the blades as necessary, until perfectly smooth. Set aside. (Note: If using a conventional blender, do it this way: Grind the chia seeds in a coffee grinder until you have a *very* fine powder. Set aside. Blend the remaining fluff ingredients in your blender until smooth. Transfer to a food processor along with the ground chia; process to blend.)

Make the crumble: In a clean food processor, pulse the walnuts, hemp seeds, lucuma, salt, coconut flour, stevia, and cinnamon until the mixture resembles bread crumbs (there shouldn't be any visible pieces of walnut). Take care not to overprocess or the oil will begin to separate out. Drizzle the vanilla and nondairy milk over the crumbs and pulse a few times to moisten the crumbs (don't process until you have a single ball; it should still be crumbly).

Make the chocolate drizzle: Bring about 2 inches (5 cm) of water to a simmer in a small pot. Place a heatproof bowl over the pot so that the bottom of the bowl doesn't touch the water. Place the cacao and coconut oil in the bowl and stir until the oil is melted. Remove from the heat and stir in the stevia and vanilla.

Assemble the parfaits: Set aside about 2 tablespoons (30 ml) of the crumble to reserve for the tops of the parfaits. Next, place about 1 tablespoon (15 ml) of unpacked crumbs in the bottom of each parfait glass. Top with about 2 tablespoons (30 ml) of the fluff, spreading it out to reach the sides of the glass. Drizzle about 2 teaspoons (10 ml) of the chocolate over the fluff. Repeat with another layer of crumbs and fluff. Crumble the reserved crumbs over the fluff and then drizzle with the remaining chocolate. Allow to firm up in the refrigerator for at least 2 to 4 hours.

Note: The drizzle becomes hard when refrigerated, so ensure that you don't cover the entire surface of the parfait with it, or you'll end up with a solid mass of chocolate you'll need to break through (not the worst thing in the world, but the parfaits are easier to eat if the fluff isn't entirely covered by the chocolate). These will keep, covered, in the refrigerator for up to 4 days. Not suitable for freezing.

Note: You can make the marshmallow fluff in a regular blender by soaking the cashews first for 4 to 6 hours in room-temperature water, then draining before use; use only ⅓ cup (80 ml) of Homemade Coconut Milk (page 99) in that case.

Note: If you find that raw cacao triggers cravings for you, use the carob option here in Stage 1.

Vanilla Ice Cream
Good for: Stage 2 and beyond

Imagine a thick, decadent, French vanilla ice cream made complex with the richness of real egg custard and vanilla beans. The synergy of pear for sweetness, macadamias for richness and just a hint of English toffee stevia for depth of flavor re-creates the best vanilla ice cream you've ever tasted in this recipe—and you don't even need an ice-cream maker to enjoy this one!

MAKES 6 TO 8 SERVINGS

1 (14-ounce [400 ml]) can full-fat coconut milk, preferably organic

⅔ cup (105 to 115 g) raw macadamia nuts or cashews

2 medium-size ripe pears, cored (no need to peel)

1 teaspoon (5 ml) vanilla powder, or 2 teaspoons (10 ml) pure vanilla extract

⅓ cup (80 ml) unsweetened almond or other nondairy milk of choice

Pinch fine sea salt

½ teaspoon (2.5 ml) SweetLeaf English Toffee—flavored pure liquid stevia, or ⅛ teaspoon (0.5 ml) pure stevia powder, or other pure liquid stevia, to taste; or ¼ cup (60 ml) coconut sugar or coconut nectar, plus more stevia to taste for stage 3 and beyond (Note: If you use the coconut nectar/sugar, your vanilla ice cream will be a light tan color!)

Optional add-ins: ¼ cup (60 ml) cacao nibs; chopped pecans or other nuts of choice; oven-dried cranberries or blueberries; chopped fresh berries; homemade chocolate or carob chips (page 205).

Line a twelve-cup muffin tin with nine silicone muffin liners. Alternatively, set out three resealable plastic bags.

Place all the ingredients, except the add-ins, in a blender and blend until perfectly smooth. Taste and adjust the sweetness level.

Divide the mixture evenly among the muffin liners or the three bags and seal the bags, pressing out any air. Place the ice cream in the freezer and chill until solid, for at least 4 hours. Once the ice cream is solid, pop it out of the muffin liners and store in resealable plastic bags until ready to use.

To make in a food processor: For two servings, take two or three of the frozen "muffins" or the contents of one plastic bag and chop into chunks (I usually cut each "muffin" into four pieces). Process until it looks like crumbs, then scrape down the sides and continue to process until the ice cream comes together smoothly. If using add-ins, add them to the processor and pulse one to three times just to incorporate. Scoop into bowls and serve immediately.

To make in an ice-cream maker: Do not freeze the ice cream in muffin cups or plastic bags first. Once the mixture is blended, pour it into your ice-cream maker and follow manufacturer's instructions. Add your choice of add-ins in the last 5 minutes of churning. Freeze and serve.

Classic Whipped Cream
Good for: all stages

This is my new go-to coconut whipped cream. Cashews increase the richness, but also the thickness, of the cream, so that it retains its shape at room temperature much longer than cream made just from the coconut "cream."

MAKES ABOUT 2 CUPS (480 ML) WHIPPED CREAM

1 (14-ounce [400 ml]) can full-fat organic coconut milk, chilled
    in the fridge for at least 24 hours
⅓ cup (55 g) raw cashews, or 2 tablespoons (30 ml) raw
    cashew butter (you can use regular cashew butter, but the
    cream won't be as firm)
2 teaspoons (10 ml) vanilla powder or pure vanilla extract
Pinch of fine sea salt
5 to 10 drops plain or vanilla stevia, or to taste

Remove the can from your refrigerator and turn it upside down. Open the can (i.e., remove what was the bottom) and pour off the thick, clear liquid there. You can save the liquid for smoothies or to use in baking.

Scoop out the thick coconut cream and place in a high-powered blender with the other ingredients (if you don't have a high-powered blender, use cashew butter instead of raw cashews). Blend until smooth, using the tamper, if necessary, to push the nuts into the blades. The mixture may liquefy somewhat while blending; this is fine. Pour into a container and refrigerate until firm, 8 hours or overnight. When ready to use, you can just scoop the cream as is or fluff it up by beating with an electric mixer or a handheld whisk for 30 seconds or so. Will keep, covered, in the refrigerator for up to 2 days.

Part III

Life After Candida

CHAPTER 14

Lifestyle Strategies for a Lifetime Without Candida

In this chapter, I address the question that each of us who's ever followed an anticandida diet ponders: Is there life after candida? (Spoiler alert: yes.)

One afternoon while in our twenties, my best friend, Robin, and I were out for a stroll on one of the first spring days of the season. You know the kind: the sun suffuses the sky with late afternoon brilliance, lawns begin to soften and emit their grassy scent, and the exuberant trilling of birds returns to the air overhead. As we snaked our way up and down the neighborhood streets, Robin unexpectedly announced that she had quit smoking. At the time, almost everyone I knew smoked cigarettes, if not full-time, then socially at parties or out to dinner with friends; I myself was still indulging in the occasional puff at the time. "I will never smoke another cigarette again," she proclaimed.

Well, I was gobsmacked. "But how can you *say* that?" I insisted, a note of panic in my voice. "How do you *know* you'll never smoke again?" I'd never been that certain about anything, not even my first love. "For as long as I live," she responded. "I just know."

There was no way I could see myself being that determined about quitting anything. It took candida, and several years on a "special" diet, for me to reach that level of conviction.

In fact, for quite some time, even as I followed the ACD to a T, I was a living example of Elisabeth Kübler-Ross's five stages of grieving as they apply to dieting. First was

Denial (I put off confirming my diagnosis because I couldn't consciously accept the situation); then Anger ("Why me? It's not fair! So-and-so eats way more sugar than I do, and *she* doesn't have candida!"); on to Bargaining ("Maybe if I am really strict this month, I'll be able to eat cake at my cousin's wedding on the weekend"); and Depression ("This is never ending. How long is this going to go on? Why am I the one who has to give up sugar?"); and finally, Acceptance ("I can take any recipe and make it ACD-friendly. As God is my witness, I will never eat sugar again").

I have no doubt that some who are battling candida will, indeed, be able to return to a diet that contains a certain amount of refined sugar, or refined flour, or alcohol, for instance, without seeing adverse effects. I am not one of those people. Because of earlier damage done to my body by years of overconsuming sugars, as well as daily consumption of junk foods, I've come to accept that my body simply can't tolerate those things. And while I may, one day, reach a point where I'd be able to partake of conventional cake, or processed foods, to a small degree—well, to be honest, I don't really want to any more, anyway. (I do still fantasize about a gin and tonic once in a while during summer months, however.)

In other words, if you need to begin this diet, some form of the ACD will likely become an ongoing proposition. No, you won't have to stick to the strictest form of the diet indefinitely, and you will certainly be able to loosen up the restrictions as you begin to feel better and heal. But it only makes sense—and is best for your health—to remain on a modified version of the diet even once the yeast has taken a hike.

For me, a lifetime anticandida plan means eating foods that don't encourage candida to grow; adapting recipes so that they contain health-promoting, and often antifungal, ingredients; and trying to adapt my home so that external factors that could contribute to the condition are also kept at bay.

So read on for tips and techniques to reduce candida, as well as other toxins that can wear down immunity, throughout your home and out in the world. These everyday precautions will help ensure that you continue to enjoy better health while on the program—and beyond.

Keeping Candida at Bay in the Home

Avoiding mold in the home is as equally important as avoiding it in your food, especially because spores can exist in the air and you won't necessarily know they're there.

(I'm not talking about deadly "black mold" in this case, though of course it's imperative to avoid that, too; I mean everyday molds and fungi that nevertheless can be harmful as well.) Keeping your house free of mold and other toxins is an important step toward ensuring that candida won't return for an encore engagement once you've cleared it out of your internal system. Once you begin to dig into the plethora of toxins that reside in most modern homes, clearing up the air and surfaces alone can become a full-time endeavor! While there are far too many possible culprits to mention here— from furniture finishing to floor coverings to kitchen containers, cosmetics, cleaners, and self-care items—some simple changes can help improve the quality of the air you breathe and decrease the daily assault on your immune system from within the home.

Bathrooms and Kitchens

Bathrooms and kitchens are notorious breeding grounds for mold, mostly because they are wet on a daily basis.

Obviously, it makes sense to keep your bathroom and kitchen as clean and dry as possible. Because direct sunlight can kill fungus and other pathogens, throw open those curtains and pull up the blinds if your rooms will be flooded with sunshine as a result.

In addition, it's important to regularly examine anything in the kitchen or bathroom that tends to remain damp over a period of time, such as your dishcloths, drain boards, or scrubbers (be they those you use to clean pots or your body in the shower).[1]

Basements

My first bout with candida occurred while I was living in a small postwar home that I'd bought at a bargain basement price. Well, you know what they say about getting what you pay for. . . .

On the day I moved out after living for three years in the house, the movers had just about finished lugging boxes from the basement. When they reached a certain spot and picked up one of many boxes of books, the bottom fell right out of the box—the cardboard was soaking wet. A huge area, perhaps a 6-foot (1.8 m) square, of the basement floor was soaked, in fact, and all of the boxes that had been resting there were ruined, stinking of mold.

MAGIC MOLD AND MILDEW CLEANER

My friend Tess Masters hails from Australia, and she swears by her mum's recipe for a natural antimold and mildew spray. I remembered her blog post about this recipe when I was writing this chapter, and she graciously agreed to let me post it here. According to Tess, this solution works wonders in bathrooms and on surfaces. As she says, "Give this solution a go and you will never touch toxic bleaches and disinfectants again!"[2]

Magic Mold and Mildew Cleaner
(courtesy of Tess Masters, http://theblendergirl.com)

½ cup (120 ml) borax
½ cup (120 ml) distilled white vinegar
2 cups (480 ml) warm water
2 teaspoons (10 ml) tea tree oil

1. Dissolve the borax and vinegar in the warm water.
2. Add the tea tree oil.
3. Pour this into a spray bottle.
4. Spray the affected areas and scrub with a brush.
5. Rinse with warm water and wipe over.
6. This is fantastic for shower curtains and shower walls.

Of course, I'd been living the entire time oblivious since I rarely went into the basement and certainly hadn't thought to systematically check beneath the boxes when everything on the surface appeared fine. Looking back, I realize I'd been breathing in moldy air likely for the entire time I lived in the house (and don't forget that a forced-air heating system, such as I had there, circulates the air everywhere). Not coincidentally, my sinus problems began shortly after I moved into that house.

Nowadays, I regularly head to the basement once a week for a quick survey and ensure there are no wet spots, moisture, moldy patches, and so on. That way, if mold does begin to develop for some reason, I'll catch it immediately and can deal with it (oh, and I've purchased plastic bins in which to store anything made of cloth or paper, too). If you have cardboard or wooden storage in the basement, be sure to keep boxes or containers away from concrete floors and walls (where they might become food for mold, as mine did).

If you use your basement as part of your living space, it's also a good idea to use smooth flooring rather than carpets, as mold loves to grow in carpeting. If you can, keep windows open or use fans to keep air flowing through the basement and to keep it well ventilated. Purchasing a dehumidifier for the basement is also a good idea (keep the relative humidity at less than 50 percent for best effect).

Other Rooms (Living Room, Bedroom, etc.)

Plants: I was surprised to learn that houseplants can be a source of mold. When the soil is kept too damp, mold grows easily and the spores can become airborne and subsequently inhaled, causing more problems for anyone with candida.[3] On the other hand, plants also consume carbon dioxide and many work as natural air filters to remove other toxins in the air, from formaldehyde to benzene and chloroform.[4] To enjoy the benefits of houseplants, refrain from overwatering your plants, to avoid mold growth, or simply change the soil once or twice a year for the same effect.

Windowsills and walls: In all rooms, check windowsills and walls for signs of mold growth; keep these areas dry and as clean as possible. Using the Magic Mold and Mildew Cleaner (page 228) works on these surfaces as well.

Linens and upholstery: When dealing with washable fabrics, such as linens or upholstery, add ½ to 1 teaspoonful (2.5 to 5 ml) of grapefruit seed extract to each load of laundry to help disinfect it and keep mold from growing.

General Advice for a Nontoxic Home

According to Lara Adler, an environmental toxins expert and certified holistic health coach, there are several steps to ensure that the general level of toxins in the home is kept to a minimum. The goal is to keep the levels low enough that your body won't become overwhelmed and trigger an overactive immune system, one of the ways candida gains a foothold (sporehold?) in the first place. Here are some simple, and a couple of more advanced, tips that anyone can employ.

Bring the outside inside. Sunshine is known to kill pathogenic organisms, which is why our elders used to hang clothes out in the sun and why a rug can be cleaned simply by being aired outside. Throw open those curtains or draw up the blinds and let the sunshine in.

According to Adler, you should also frequently open your windows, as the interior air is often more polluted than the external air; all the chemicals and outgassing that happens from sprays, cleansers, and so on remain indoors without any discernable route out. Open the windows and give those critters an escape hatch.[5]

Leave the outside, outside. While air is one thing, dirt, debris, and exterior chemicals are another. Adler suggests removing your shoes at the door every time you enter the house. That way, you won't be tracking in chemical residues or other toxins that can become embedded in your carpets without any way out.[6] I keep a pair of "indoor-only" shoes by the door so I can change into them as soon as I get home.

When it comes to cleansers, be old-fashioned. When I was a kid, my dad would institute "cleanup days" on his day off from work (I know, the guy really needed a hobby). I remember being amazed that he'd clean the windows and mirrors the way his own grandmother had, with a piece of newspaper and a spray bottle of regular ole vinegar. Those windows were clearer and more sparkly than when my mother used her favorite blue spray.

Adler confirmed that my dad's approach is still the best one: whenever possible, go back to the most basic, natural cleaning and self-care products you can find. The simplest are vinegar and baking soda, which, individually or mixed together, can take care of 90 percent of your cleaning needs. And while some recent studies have suggested that we don't need antibacterial soaps and wipes to kill inhospitable organisms,[7] if you're concerned about them, you can always add a few drops of antibacterial essential oils (such as thyme, cinnamon, lemon, or clove), both to provide a scent and to add antibacterial properties, a natural function of these oils.[8]

Avoid synthetic packaging and products. Adler believes the one most important step you can take to reduce overall toxic load in the kitchen is to shun plastic wrap and containers that come in contact with food, as those molecules can easily be absorbed into the food (she suggests switching to glass). In addition, note that many canned goods are lined with BPA (bisphenol-A), a highly toxic compound that can also be absorbed into the food inside. Look for BPA-free cans.[9]

These rules also apply to personal care products and cosmetics. Adler's best tip here is to look for the word *fragrance* on the product, as this invariably indicates synthetic or chemical ingredients.[10] Look for products that contain natural ingredients you can recognize.

Finally, be wary of air fresheners, which are not only synthetic but not necessary. Keep your home clean and open windows regularly for the best air freshener possible![11]

Keeping Candida at Bay When You're Out in the World

Social Situations

Balancing your diet with the desire to socialize can sometimes seem like a challenge, but it is eminently doable! With a little planning and some flexibility, you'll find that you can still attend social situations, celebrate birthdays with family, or celebrate at the office Christmas party without ruining your progress on the anticandida diet. The most important aspect of these situations, in the end, is your own attitude about them. As I said earlier, *different* doesn't necessarily equate with *negative*, so enjoy your healthy foods and have fun!

Here are some practical steps you can take to ensure that you enjoy the event while still feasting with the rest of the crowd.

Consult in advance. When you first receive any invitation, give the host or hostess a call and explain the situation to see if whoever is overseeing the food is amenable to including something you can eat. (If you're comfortable with it, you could even ask the person to save any packaging for you so you can read the ingredients and ensure that everything is "candida-safe.")

Oftentimes, my friends will set aside a serving of a recipe, say, a salad, for me before adding dressing so that they don't have to whip up an entirely new dish on my account; this way, I'm able to consume the "same" salad as everyone else without drawing attention to my plate. Alternatively, offer to help prepare the food and set aside something that you can eat beforehand. If that kind of compromise isn't possible or practical, then be sure to bring your own (next point).

Bring your own. One of Andrea's tricks that I regularly employ is to bring both a savory and a sweet dish to social gatherings to ensure I blend in with everyone else. Doing so guarantees that I'll never find myself without something "safe" to eat, and my plate need never appear empty. While others snack on appetizers or the main meal, even if there's virtually nothing I can eat on offer, I can turn to my savory dish. And during dessert, I enjoy the sweet recipe I brought.

I try to take along a dish big enough to share with everyone (or, in a large group, six to ten servings). On more than one occasion, my friends and their children have been curious enough to try my meal and were pleasantly surprised at how tasty it is! These days, they request their favorite desserts, knowing their kids will devour them.

If all else fails, keep your mouth shut. There will be times when, despite your best efforts, you'll find yourself in situations where there is little to nothing you can eat. In these cases, I've found that the best practice is to keep my mouth shut—literally and figuratively. No, I don't mean that you shouldn't continue to chat and enjoy conversations, but, where food is concerned, if you're in doubt, play it safe and simply don't eat it. It's highly unlikely that you'll faint from hunger even if you have to wait until you get back home to eat something ACD-friendly (or, if you're fairly certain before you leave that the culinary landscape will be sparse at your destination, then grab a "safe" bite before you go).

I have found that it's generally unhelpful to reprimand a host or hostess who forgot about or simply botched your food; most people wish to be accommodating but may not know how. If someone is genuinely attempting to be helpful, I thank them and move on. The next time, I bring something of my own with me.

Focus on what really counts. Finally, while it may be true that in our culture, food is often the centerpiece of any social gathering, don't lose sight of the real reason you've all come together: to socialize and interact with friends and/or family. If you've had a little snack before you arrived, or if you brought at least two items you can eat, then your menu will be covered, and it doesn't really matter if you don't partake of any other foods at the table. The less I focus on my plate, the less my friends feel awkward, too—and we can all enjoy a pleasant social experience together.

Restaurants

Most restaurants these days are accustomed to special requests from diners with allergies or other food restrictions. If you think of your anticandida diet as simply one more similar special request, it becomes much easier to seek out and ask for what you need to dine comfortably and enjoyably.

Where to go? Living near Toronto, I'm blessed with access to one of the most multicultural cities in the world, which also means there is a vast array of multicultural restaurants from which to choose.

I've found that certain types of cuisine are much more anticandida diet–friendly than others. As a rule, some of the best ACD-friendly dishes can be found in Asian, Mexican, Indian, Middle Eastern, and vegan restaurants, where menus offer a good selection of simple or vegetable-only dishes; some health food stores may have in-house cafés as well. However, be aware that many Chinese restaurants still use MSG in their foods. In addition, many sauces contain sugar or flour; and soy products (e.g., soy sauce) tend to be GMO (genetically modified), unless organic. Be vigilant about asking questions to ensure that the food is safe to eat!

Expect to pay more. In general, upscale restaurants are more accommodating, not only because they are more customer-oriented but also because their food is more often made à la minute (from scratch) and can be altered without unsettling an entire kitchen. The quality of the food in an upscale restaurant will also be better, and your chances of finding something organic increase.

Call in advance. Call in advance so the establishment has a chance to prepare for you. This will also give you an opportunity to explain your dietary restrictions and see if it is able to accommodate you. If you can, aim to speak with the restaurant manager or head chef, as this is the one who'll be planning and handling the food or has the power to approve a change in the regular menu.

Ask three times. I always ask about my meal three separate times: first, when I call in advance; next, when I'm seated and order my meal; and finally, right before I eat. Three times may seem like overkill, but remember that, ultimately, no one cares as much about your diet as you do.

On one occasion, a friend and I dined at a local Chinese restaurant. I called in advance to ensure that it had a gluten-free option for me and was assured that it did. When we arrived at the restaurant, however, I noticed that the dish the server recommended contained soy sauce. When I inquired whether it was gluten-free, she had no idea. I asked to see the bottle and, sure enough, the chef was using regular soy sauce that contained wheat—*and sugar*! In the end, the chef prepared the dish for me without any sauce, but I learned my lesson. In a case like that, it may actually be useful to refer to your dietary restrictions in terms of allergies, as most restaurants are more careful to accommodate you in that case.

Keep it simple. If you aren't sure about the quality or ingredients of the food at a particular establishment, keeping the choice as simple as possible is the best course of action. Order a salad without dressing, plain steamed vegetables, or steamed rice if in doubt; almost every restaurant will have those items on hand.

Avoid the rush. Arriving either before or after the dinnertime rush will ensure that staff isn't too busy to accommodate your requests. Your waitperson and chef alike will be much more inclined to listen and attempt to meet your needs if they're not distracted by crowds of other diners all vying for their attention.

Traveling

If you travel for work, or if you have a vacation scheduled and are concerned about whether you'll be able to maintain the diet, there are some precautions to take to ensure that you'll still be well fed away from home.

Keep it homey. If you're staying for any length of time in another city, many hotels offer "efficiency" rooms with a small refrigerator, stove, and so on. It's always best if you can cook your own meals and keep your own food on hand. Even if your stay is just overnight, call in advance and request a refrigerator in the room so that you can keep homemade snacks and breakfasts at the ready.

Bring your own. After I'd been on the diet for a while and had reintroduced fruits, my husband and I took a short trip to New York. I knew that the Big Apple, of all cities, would likely be home to at least several restaurants where I could comfortably eat. Because it's a relatively short flight from Toronto, I didn't bother to pack any snacks as I knew I'd be able to buy something at the local Whole Foods or health food store once we landed.

As it turned out, we were required to be at the airport at 6 a.m. After scanning the airport café menu for some ACD–friendly foods, I realized that the only foods even vaguely acceptable were fresh fruit cups; but even those were made exclusively of melons (high in mold) and grapes (far too high in sugar). I ordered a green tea and waited for lunch. Subsequently, our flight was delayed; once we landed, it took two hours to reach the hotel from the airport; in the end, it was close to 6 p.m. before I ate anything.

I learned my lesson and never (ever) travel anywhere without some homemade food on hand. Even for a quick trip downtown, I ensure I've got a bag of mixed nuts and seeds in the car in case I'm stuck in traffic or don't get home as soon as anticipated. That way, I avoid the risk of buying something I shouldn't eat so as to assuage my hunger.

Some of my travel staples include ACD-Friendly Grain-Free Granola (page 123), Almost Instant Grain-Free Breakfast Porridge (page 127), "Sour Cream and Onion" Kale Chips (page 139), and Sweet and Spicy Roasted Chickpeas (page 138), which all hold up well when packed.

Do your research. Spend some time on Google before you book your vacation to ensure there will be food for you once you arrive at your destination. It's also a good idea to check for nearby health food stores or supermarkets likely to carry healthy foods and buy some raw ingredients for ACD–friendly snacks and light meals. With a bit of advance prep, you can head out and truly enjoy your time away from home!

Yeast Assessment Form

Name: Age: Sex: Date:

Please list your most major signs or symptoms in the order of importance:
1.   2.   3.   4.   5.

Please circle the appropriate number for each of the questions in sections 1–4 below.
0 = not an issue   1 = present but manageable   2 = distressing   3 = miserable

SECTION 1				
My bowels do not seem to empty completely.	0	1	2	3
I experience lower abdominal pain that is relieved by passing gas.	0	1	2	3
My bowels alternate between constipation and diarrhea.	0	1	2	3
I regularly experience constipation.	0	1	2	3
I eliminate less than one time a day.	0	1	2	3
I regularly experience diarrhea.	0	1	2	3
I eliminate more than three times a day.	0	1	2	3
My gas and poop tend to be foul smelling.	0	1	2	3
My poop can be "sticky" or not fully formed on a regular basis.	0	1	2	3
My belly can bloat or swell easily after eating.	0	1	2	3
I experience abdominal pain.	0	1	2	3
I sometimes see undigested food in my stool.	0	1	2	3
I get an uncomfortable sense of fullness during or after meals.	0	1	2	3
I get heartburn after eating or when lying down.	0	1	2	3
I use antacids.	0	1	2	3
I sometimes experience pain or tenderness on my left side, under my rib cage.	0	1	2	3
I am hungry all the time, and quickly after eating (within an hour or two).	0	1	2	3
I'm sensitive to smells, such as smoke or perfume.	0	1	2	3
My symptoms worsen in damp or muggy conditions.	0	1	2	3
Section 1 score: Add up the numbers that you scored in Section 1, see where it falls within the ranges below, and mark that number (1, 2, or 3) as your Total Section 1 Score. **0–12 = 1 12–24 = 2 24 or higher = 3 Total Section 1 Score**				

SECTION 2

I seem to have a reaction to many foods I eat (skin irritations, digestive disturbances, or changes in focus or mood).	0	1	2	3
I often cannot tell what foods I'm reacting to.	0	1	2	3
At times I experience aches and pains throughout my body.	0	1	2	3
I seem to have intolerances to sugars and starches.	0	1	2	3
I often experience itchy skin, rashes or hives, bumpy skin or rough skin, or have a history of thrush.	0	1	2	3
I have vaginal burning or itching or unusual discharge.	0	1	2	3
I experience frequent urination or burning when urinating.	0	1	2	3
I experience PMS.	0	1	2	3
I have joint and/or muscle pain.	0	1	2	3
I experience anal itching.	0	1	2	3
I've had more than one yeast infection in the last three years.	0	1	2	3
I have nail or skin fungus (ringworm, athlete's foot, fungal skin rash, etc.).	0	1	2	3
My ears are itchy.	0	1	2	3
Section 2 score: Add up the numbers that you scored in Section 2, see where it falls within the ranges below and mark that number (1, 2, or 3) as your Total Section 2 Score. **0–10 = 1 10–20 = 2 20 or higher = 3 Total Section 2 Score**				

SECTION 3

It's difficult for me to lose weight, no matter what I do.	0	1	2	3
My hair is thinning and is falling out.	0	1	2	3
I crave sweets throughout the day.	0	1	2	3
Eating sweets does not relieve my cravings for sugar.	0	1	2	3
I often want sweets at the end of a meal.	0	1	2	3
I'm irritable or lightheaded if I miss a meal.	0	1	2	3
I rely on coffee (or chocolate) to get me through the day.	0	1	2	3
I experience fatigue after meals.	0	1	2	3
I rarely stay asleep throughout the night.	0	1	2	3
I crave salt.	0	1	2	3
I am slow to get moving in the morning.	0	1	2	3
I can barely keep my eyes open in the afternoon.	0	1	2	3
I have experienced reproductive issues.	0	1	2	3
Section 3 score: Add up the numbers that you scored in Section 3, see where it falls within the ranges below and mark that number (1, 2, or 3) as your Total Section 3 Score. **0–12 = 1 12–24 = 2 24 or higher = 3 Total Section 3 Score**				

continues →

SECTION 4				
I sometimes feel shaky or experience the jitters.	0	1	2	3
I experience anxiety or depression.	0	1	2	3
I'm agitated easily.	0	1	2	3
I am nervous and emotional.	0	1	2	3
I am more forgetful than in the past.	0	1	2	3
I often feel foggy-brained, spacey, or lightheaded.	0	1	2	3
It's difficult for me to concentrate or stay on task.	0	1	2	3
My vision is blurred.	0	1	2	3
I experience headaches.	0	1	2	3
I sometimes get dizzy when standing up.	0	1	2	3
I have balance problems.	0	1	2	3
Section 4 score: Add up the numbers that you scored in Section 4, see where it falls within the ranges below and mark that number (1, 2, or 3) as your Total Section 4 Score. **0–12 = 1 12–24 = 2 24 or higher = 3** **Total Section 4 Score**				

Please circle the appropriate response for each of the questions in section 5 below.

SECTION 5			
I consume ___ alcoholic beverages per week.	0–3	3–5	5+
I currently eat refined sugar.	N	Y	
I currently eat refined grains or flours.	N	Y	
I currently drink regular or diet soda.	N	Y	
My stress level per week would rate as follows (0 = none; 5 = high).	0–3	3–5	5+
I have taken antibiotics for one month or longer or have repeatedly taken short-course antibiotics.	N	Y	
I have taken prednisone or other cortico-steroids for one month or longer.	N	Y	
I have taken birth control pills for one year or longer.	N	Y	
Score +2 points for each circle in a gray column **Total Score for section 5**			

Total Score for Sections 1 through 5 (add up final scores from each section) _____

  0–4   *Mild & Manageable:* You're in good shape and tracking the stages will most certainly support your health.

  5–8   *Moderate & Maleable:* Get a handle on it now and you may move quickly through the stages.

  9–14   *Distressing & Persistent:* Reassess every three months to see whether you have found some relief and can move on.

  14+   *Chronic & Feeling Miserable:* You may need to stay at Stage 1 for a longer duration to begin to experience results; hang in there!

ACKNOWLEDGMENTS

I can think of nothing more rewarding than being able to write a book on a topic so close to my heart, and I feel privileged to have this opportunity to share it with so many of you; for that, I am truly thankful. There are also many people to thank for ultimately leading me here and helping me along the way, and I'm grateful to them all. (And to those of you not listed here, please know that your input was no less appreciated).

To the readers of my site, rickiheller.com as well as those of you I've met through social media, talks, or other events, thank you for your continued support, feedback, comments, and enthusiasm. I could never have guessed when I started my blog that it would eventually come to touch the lives of so many people, and I am grateful every day for the relationships created because of it. I hope this book speaks to you as well.

To Andrea Nakayama, my sister from another mister: whatever prompted you to send that tweet and initiate our first collaboration, I am eternally grateful. Your knowledge and expertise as a practitioner and your insight, sensitivity, and emotional intelligence as a friend are constant sources of inspiration to me. Thank you for making the time to contribute some of your genius to this book, without which it wouldn't have been half as good (nor as much fun to write). I adore you.

To Renée Sedliar, if I had conjured my ideal editor, I couldn't have dreamt up anyone as amazing as you. Thank you for your constant support, your always accurate eye, your passion for and understanding of my vision for this book, your diplomacy. Your ability to take my text and somehow magically re-vision it enabled this book to be the very best it could be. I am *your* biggest fan.

To the team at Da Capo: Thank you to Cisca Schreefel for expertly overseeing this project to its completion, to Iris Bass for your detailed and diligent copyedits (and sorry, still no turnip), to Alex Camlin for bringing the cover to life; to Timm Bryson for the book's layout; as well as to Claire Ivett for your expert assistance. Thanks also to proofreader, Lori Lewis, and indexer, Doug Easton.

To Kate Cassaday at Harper Collins Canada, thanks for your review and input on the manuscript and for helping to shape its final form.

To my agent, Marilyn Allen, eternal thanks for championing this book and finding its home at Da Capo, and for your continued support and friendship.

To Nicole Axworthy, thank you for taking on this project when you had so many others already on the go, and for making it work within my crazy schedule. And most important, thank you for making my food look so mouthwateringly good!

To Cristina Favreau, thank you for your always impeccable work, your incredible attention to detail, for consistently knowing what needs to be done long before I do, and for embodying excellence and professionalism. I am so thrilled and honored to have you in my corner and look forward to more years as colleagues and friends.

To the book's incredible recipe testers, thank you for the hours spent in the kitchen diligently testing and retesting recipes. Your devotion to this project, your many insights, suggestions, and feedback improved and perfected these recipes. Andria Barrett, Barrie Allen, Courtney Blair, Denise McFadden, Emma Potts, Holly Sue Brady, Irene Prasad, Jennifer Ward, Jesse Schelew, Johanna Monk, Karina Minchin, Katja Haudenhuyse, Kelli Roberts, and Michele Silvester, thanks so much.

To Brigitte Fiorino, thank you for your incredibly conscientious and detail-oriented research that helped to support the details in the book.

To Alison Shefler, Barbara Freeman, Bev Verstege, Carla Flamer, Deborah Salsberg, Ela Borenstein, Judith Carson, Maria-Elena Alvarez, Michelle Spring, Robin Flamer, and Rosalyn Benatar, you've been there with me all along as I've navigated this sometimes wacky diet, accommodating my dietary needs along the way, sharing my food, and supporting the journey in myriad ways. I'm so grateful for your friendship.

To Alisa Fleming, Dreena Burton, and Tess Masters, thank you for making the leap beyond the blogs. I am ever grateful for your friendship, your wisdom, and your humor, and for all those phone calls in which you supported me and talked through the process when insecurities and hurdles surfaced (as they tend to do).

To Adrienne Urban, Allyson Kramer, Alta Mantsch, Amie Valpone, Amy Green, Carol Kicinski, Cara Lyons, Catherine Kleiser, Cheryl Harris, Christy Morgan, Gena Hamshaw, Hallie Klecker, Heather Nicholds, Jaime Karpovich, Kristina Sloggett, Jennifer Fugo, JL Fields, Julie Waterhouse, Lexie Croft, Lisa Pitman, Kim Lutz, Kim Maes, Lisa Cantkier, Maggie Savage, Marly McMillen-Beelman, Nava Atlas, Shirley Braden, Stephanie Weaver, Susan Baker, Tess Challis, and Wendy Polisi: thank you for populating my workdays with engaging conversations, humor, and your collective wisdom. I'm lucky to have colleagues and friends with whom I love working so much.

To Kathleen Kerr, Eric Marsden, Alexandra Hurtado, and Rosemary FitzGerald, thanks for your advice, assistance and kind support throughout my personal journey with candida.

To the experts who generously offered their time in interviews and provided key information about other approaches to candida, many thanks to Tarilee Cornish, Samantha Brody, Michelle Weir, and Pamela Frank; and a special thanks to Lara Adler for sharing your expertise on detoxifying the home.

To Shari, thanks for the many fun debates on allopathic-vs.-alternative medicine. (Okay, not really. But the rest of the conversations were fun.) Thank you for always being there when I called (and for answering even if I woke you up). I like the way this friendship is going.

To Cameron, thank you for your calm acceptance, no matter what, even when I disappeared for most of the day and for months at a time, because you knew how important it was to me. Thank you for still being here. Thank you for one mood, all the time. I love you.

Finally, thank you to Elsie and Chaser for being a daily source of joy. Woof and play bows.
—Ricki Heller

To Ricki Heller, who's become a dear friend, a trusted confidante, a winning collaborator and, of course, an inspiration in my kitchen, for the insight to put this book together and the generosity to ask me to join forces with her.

To Andie Jones, Megan Liebmann, Caroline Stahlschmidt, Jennifer Baum, and Katie Pugh—the stellar Replenish PDX Nutrition Team—for their continued support, clinical wisdom, manuscript review, and Questionnaire testing.

To the remainder of the Replenish PDX team, especially Brion Oliver, for the hard work and tremendous ability to hold down the fort, even while I'm busy writing.

To all our clients and customers who teach me every day and in every way about the nuances, complexities, and individual expression of symptoms, and for their stealth pursuit of the protocols and practices that will best serve their health.

To Renée Sedliar of Perseus Books, for her compassionate editing and patience. And Erin Donley for her personal copyediting.

And to the best kid on the block, my son Gilbert, for his willingness to try any recipe under the sun (as long as it's not a "bar"). So many people around the globe are served in their health crisis because of your maturity, support, and understanding.

—Andrea Nakayama

RESOURCES

BOOKS: BOOKS WITH USEFUL INFORMATION ABOUT CANDIDA OR NATURAL HEALING

Balch, Phyllis. *Prescription for Nutritional Healing.* New York: Avery, 2000.

Coulston, Ann M., and Carol J. Boushey, eds. *Nutrition in the Prevention and Treatment of Disease.* Amsterdam: Elsevier/AP, 2013.

Gates, Donna. *The Body Ecology Diet: Recovering Your Health and Rebuilding Your Immunity.* Bogart, Georgia: B.E.D. Publications, 2007.

Kjaer, Joanna, and Gill Jacobs. *Beat Candida Through Diet: A Complete Dietary Programme for Sufferers of Candidiasis.* London: Vermilion, 1997.

Levin, Warren, MD, and Fran Gare, ND. *Beyond the Yeast Connection.* Laguna Beach, CA: Basic Health, 2013.

Martin, Jeanne Marie, and Zoltan Rona, MD. *The Complete Candida Yeast Guidebook*, 2nd ed. Roseville, CA: Prima Health, 2000.

Nichols, Trent W., and Nancy Faass, eds. *Optimal Digestive Health: A Complete Guide.* Rochester, VT: Healing Arts Press, 2005.

Pitchford, Paul. *Healing with Whole Foods.* North Atlantic Books. Berkeley, CA: 2002.

Sanderson, Ian M., MD, and W. Allan Walker, *Development of the Gastrointestinal Tract*, vol. 1. Shelton, CT: PMPH-USA, 2000.

USEFUL WEBSITES AND BLOGS

Rickiheller.com (Ricki's site)

Replenishpdx.com (Andrea's site)

Wholeapproach.com (candida-specific)

Mercola.com (general health information)

FOOD SOURCES

Alive & Healing: tempeh (www.aliveandhealing.com)

Almond Breeze: unsweetened almond milk

Amazon: carries many of the brands listed here (amazon.com)

Bob's Red Mill: whole grains, chickpea, and Garfava flour (bobsredmill.com)

Eden Foods: sea vegetables (arame, dulse, nori); canned goods (non-BPA cans) (edenfoods.com)

Frontier Natural Products: herbs and spices (frontiercoop.com)

Growing Naturals: Pea protein, rice protein powders (growingnaturals.com)

iherb.com: good selection of organic and dried goods, spices, herbs, and supplements

Maine Coast Sea Vegetables: dulse, nori, other sea vegetables (seaveg.com/shop)

Manitoba Harvest: hemp seeds, hemp protein powder (manitobaharvest.com)

Mountain Rose Herbs: bulk herbs/spices (mountainroseherbs.com)

Native Forest: coconut milk (edwardandsons.com/native_shop_coconut.itml)

Navitas Naturals: seeds (chia, flax, hemp); cacao (nibs, powder), lucuma, yacon syrup (navitasnaturals.com)

NOW Foods: psyllium, flavored stevia (nowfoods.com)

NuNaturals: pure liquid stevia, stevia powder, stevia syrups, lo han guo (nunaturals.com)

Nutiva: Coconut oil, coconut flour, hemp seeds, hemp protein, chia seeds (nutiva.com)

Organic Traditions: raw cacao, stevia leaf powder, chia, hemp (yourorganicsources.com/)

Simply Organic: herbs and spices (simplyorganic.com)

SunWarrior: rice protein, pea protein powders (sunwarrior.com)

SweetLeaf Stevia: flavored pure liquid stevia (sweetleaf.com)

Tropical Traditions: organic coconut oil (www.tropicaltraditions.com)

Vitacost.com: good selection of organic and dried goods, spices, herbs, and supplements

Vitasave.ca: good selection of organic and dried goods, spices, herbs, and supplements

NOTES

INTRODUCTION
1. Hyman, Mark, MD. *The Blood Sugar Solution.* New York: Little, Brown and Company, 2012.
2. Kessler, David, MD. *The End of Overeating.* New York and Pennsylvania: Rodale, 2010.

CHAPTER 2: CORNERSTONES OF THE ANTICANDIDA DIET: INTRODUCING THE 4 D'S
1. http://drbenkim.com/full-body-cleanse.htm.
2. http://www.naturalnews.com/027454_cabbage_ulcers.html.
3. Quoted in http://www.naturalnews.com/027454_cabbage_ulcers.html.
4. http://foodmatters.tv/articles-1/the-benefits-of-soaking-nuts-and-seeds.
5. http://www.draxe.com/4-steps-to-heal-leaky-gut-and-autoimmune-disease/.
6. http://articles.mercola.com/sites/articles/archive/2012/05/12/dr-campbell-mcbride-on-gaps.aspx.
7. http://www.vegetarian.org.uk/campaigns/fish/.
8. http://news.nationalpost.com/2013/02/13/organic-foods-gm/.
9. http://www.latimes.com/science/la-sci-organic-foods-20140715-story.html.
10. http://articles.mercola.com/sites/articles/archive/2012/08/07/genetically-engineered-foods-hazards.aspx.
11. http://www.ewg.org/foodnews/guide.php?key=40410153.
12. http://www.med.nyu.edu/content?ChunkIID=90869.
13. http://www.niaid.nih.gov/topics/foodallergy/understanding/pages/quickfacts.aspx.
14. According to environmental medicine expert Dr. Walter Crinnion, there is no better way to detoxify.
15. http://www.patient.co.uk/doctor/jarisch-herxheimer-reaction.
16. Levin, Warren, MD, and Fran Gare, ND. *Beyond the Yeast Connection.* Laguna Beach, CA: Basic Health, 2013.
17. http://articles.mercola.com/sites/articles/archive/2012/05/12/dr-campbell-mcbride-on-gaps.aspx.
18. Gates, Donna. *Body Ecology Diet*, 10th ed. Bogart, Georgia: B.E.D. Publications, 2007.

19. Kabat-Zinn, Jon. *Full Catastrophe Living.* New York: Dell Publishing, 1990.

20. http://www.emmaseppala.com/10-science-based-reasons-start-meditating-today-infographic /#.UyJc4YVrdAR.

21. Ozbay, Fatih, MD, Douglas C. Johnson, PhD, Eleni Dimoulas, PhD, C. A. Morgan, III, MD, MA, Dennis Charney, MD, and Steven Southwick, MD. "Social Support and Resilience to Stress." *Psychiatry* 4, no. 5 (May 2007): 35–40. Retrieved from http://www.ncbi.nlm.nih.gov/pmc/articles/PMC2921311/.

22. http://pets.webmd.com/ss/slideshow-pets-improve-your-health.

23. Csikszentmihalyi, Mihaly. *Flow.* New York: Harper Perennial Modern Classics, 2008.

24. http://www.ted.com/talks/kelly_mcgonigal_how_to_make_stress_your_friend.

Chapter 3: Rebalancing Your Body Through Food and Lifestyle: The ACD Plan

1. Pitchford, Paul. *Healing with Whole Foods,* 3rd ed. Berkeley, CA: North Atlantic Books, 2002,

2. http://articles.mercola.com/sites/articles/archive/2012/02/01/is-this-one-of-natures-most -powerful-detoxification-tools.aspx.

3. http://articles.mercola.com/sites/articles/archive/2010/09/18/soy-can-damage-your-health.aspx.

4. http://www.theglobeandmail.com/life/health-and-fitness/ask-a-health-expert/so-really-is-soy -good-or-bad/article595071/; http://www.huffingtonpost.com/neal-barnard-md/settling-the-soy -controve_b_453966.html.

5. http://www.webmd.com/food-recipes/news/20110207/is-chocolate-the-next-super-food.

6. http://forum.wholeapproach.com/topic/caffeine-and-cocoa-question.

7. Gates, Donna. *The Body Ecology Diet.* Bogart, Georgia: B.E.D. Publications, 2007, 84.

8. Ibid., 68.

9. Levin, Warren M. MD, and Fran Gare, ND. *Beyond the Yeast Connection: A How-to Guide to Curing Candida and Other Yeast-Related Conditions.* Laguna Beach, CA: 2013.

10. http://www.wholeapproach.com.

11. http://www.foodreference.com/html/mold-on-food.html.

12. http://www.foodsafetywatch.org/factsheets/aflatoxins/.

13. http://growingnaturals.com/products/pea-proteins/.

14. "Antifungal Agents vs. Boric Acid for Treating Chronic Mycotic Vulvovaginitis." http://www .ncbi.nlm.nih.gov/pubmed/1941801.

15. Pitchford, Paul. *Healing with Whole Foods*, 3rd ed. Berkeley, CA: North Atlantic Books, 2002.

16. http://www.naturalnews.com/038670_heavy_metals_chelation_foods.html.

17. Ibid.

Chapter 4: Strategies for a Successful Anticandida Diet

1. http://www.stress.org/holmes-rahe-stress-inventory/.

2. McGonigal, Kelly. *The Willpower Instinct.* New York: Penguin Group, 2012.

Chapter 5: In the Kitchen: Stocking Your ACD Pantry and Ingredient Substitutions

1. http://blog.bobsredmill.com/gluten-free/guar-gum-vs-xanthan-gum/.

2. http://www.namastefoods.com/qa/.

3. http://www.glycemicindex.com/foodSearch.php.

4. http://owndoc.com/candida-albicans/mushrooms-fungi-molds-candida/.

5. http://www.drjohntafel.com/?page_id=619.

6. http://www.anapsid.org/cnd/diffdx/marinkovitchapp.html.

7. http://www.urthpro.com/blog/the-mold-help-diet-foods-to-avoid.

Chapter 14: Lifestyle Strategies for a Lifetime Without Candida

1. http://www.naturalnutrition.co.za/articles/chronic-diseases/treating-candidiasis/.

2. http://healthyblenderrecipes.com/recipes/homemade_eco_green_natural_mold_and_mildew_cleaner.

3. http://www.naturalnutrition.co.za/articles/chronic-diseases/treating-candidiasis/.

4. http://www.healthline.com/health-slideshow/air-purifying-plants#6.

5. Lara Adler telephone interview, March 18, 2014.

6. Ibid.

7. http://blogs.scientificamerican.com/guest-blog/2011/07/05/scientists-discover-that-antimicrobial-wipes-and-soaps-may-be-making-you-and-society-sick/.

8. Lara Adler telephone interview, March 18, 2014.

9. Ibid.

10. Ibid.

11. Ibid.

ABOUT THE AUTHORS

Ricki Heller, RHN, PhD, is a holistic nutritionist and author of the Amazon best seller *Naturally Sweet and Gluten-Free: 100 Allergy-Friendly Vegan Desserts* and the best-selling *Sweet Freedom: Desserts You'll Love Without Wheat, Eggs, Dairy or Refined Sugar*, one of three cookbooks recommended by Ellen DeGeneres on her website. Ricki also runs the popular blog ricki heller.com, where she has shared almost eight hundred recipes and articles about candida and living sugar-free. She is also associate editor for *Simply Gluten-Free* magazine and has written for numerous other publications, including *Allergic Living, Living Without* (now called *Gluten-Free & More*), *Clean Eating, VegNews*, and others. She appears frequently on Toronto-area television and at various health expos and conferences. Ricki lives in Vaughan, Ontario, with her husband and two Lab–border collie–cross dogs.

Functional nutritionist, educator, and speaker **Andrea Nakayama** is the founder of two global nutrition institutes, Replenish PDX and Holistic Nutrition Lab, where health-care practitioners and awakened individuals learn how to effectively care for others and take full ownership over their own health. After the loss of her young husband to a brain tumor in 2002, Andrea's dedication to personalized "food as medicine" skyrocketed into the practice she has today, which includes five nutritionists and a host of online programs. A master at simplifying and explaining why we hurt, how we heal, and what foods to eat, Andrea's been featured in *O, The Oprah Magazine*, Martha Stewart's *Whole Living*, and numerous online conferences and summits. Andrea also serves as the in-house nutrition expert for several organizations. She holds CNE and CNC certifications from Bauman College and a CHHC from the Institute of Integrative Nutrition, and is working toward a master of science degree in human nutrition and functional medicine (MSHMFM).

INDEX